TALK DIRTY

FRENCH

ALEXIS MUNIER & EMMANUEL TICHELLI

Avon, Massachusetts

Published by
Adams Media, a division of F+W Media, Inc.
57 Littlefield Street, Avon, MA 02322
www.adamsmedia.com

ISBN-13: 978-1-59869-665-3
ISBN-10: 1-59869-665-3

Printed in the United States of America.

10 9 8 7 6 5 4 3 2

Library of Congress Cataloging-in-Publication Data
is available from the publisher.

This publication is designed to provide accurate and authoritative information with regard to the subject matter covered. It is sold with the unders-
tanding that the publisher is not engaged in rendering legal, accounting, or
other professional advice. If legal advice or other expert assistance is required, the services of a competent professional person should be sought.
—From a *Declaration of Principles* jointly adopted by a Committee of the
American Bar Association and a Committee of Publishers and Associations

Many of the designations used by manufacturers and sellers to distinguish
their product are claimed as trademarks. Where those designations appear
in this book and Adams Media was aware of a trademark claim, the designations have been printed with initial capital letters.

Interior photos ©iStockphoto.com/Norma Zaro and Valerie Loiseleux.
Interior illustrations ©iStockphoto.com/Matt Knannlein.

This book is available at quantity discounts for bulk purchases.
For information, please call 1-800-289-0963.

CONTENTS

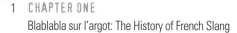

To my belle-maman Paula, whose American slang i'm just beginning to understand.

—ALEXIS MUNIER

To my belle-maman Rita, whose French slang i've understood from the beginning.

—EMMANUEL TICHELLI

Acknowledgments

A big thank you to the French and English speakers who got down and dirty for this book: Véronique Begué, Naomi Yamaguchi, Gregory Bergman, Nadia Cescon, Toby Ernberg, Jacques Bogh, Frédéric Heuer, Nicolas Verraires, Frédéric Scheidecker, Daniel Frauchiger, Giovanni Moscioni, Shamsa Abdulrasak, Jennifer Sem, Daliha Essoudi, Bruno Voirol, Matthieu Zellweger, Andrès Pasquier, Ismet Terki, Yves Ducrey, and the Tichellis.

We can't forget our language teachers and foreign penpals, who inspired us to continue learning *français* and *anglais*: Geneviève Murisier, Laurel Branam, Sarah Niles, Jeffrey Mehlman, Marie-Claude Moix, and Bénédicte Breton.

Last but not least, thanks to our publisher, Adams Media, and their stellar team including wonder woman Paula Munier, her sidekick Brendan O'Neill, editor Katrina Schroeder, and excellent French speaker (though you'd never know by his name) copyeditor Chuck Brandstater.

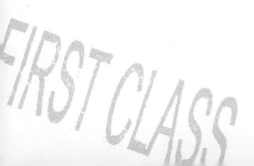

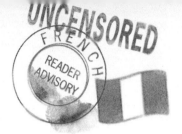

DISCLAIMER

All entries come with sample sentences as well

as common use and literal translations with the

exception of the dirtiest of the dirty.

You'll know them by

XXX: Too Dirty to Translate.

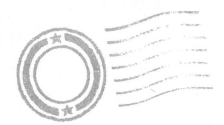

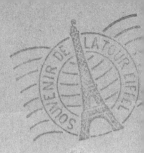

CHAPTER ONE

Blablabla sur l'argot:
The History of French slang

Dirty French didn't happen overnight. Over the course of nearly 2,000 years, French itself has evolved from Latin into the language it is today. When Latin-speaking Romans colonized France in the first century BC, their tongue was subject to variations and modifications, the result of both being far from home and interacting with the Celtic tribes in the area. By the time the Roman Empire's frontiers collapsed in the fifth century, the Latin spoken in Gaul, as France was then known, was cut off from the Latin spoken in Rome. This separation led to the birth of the French language. But several more recent reasons are behind the evolution of what we call textbook French into what we affectionately know as Dirty French.

The French colonial empire, known as *la Métropole,* was second only to the British Empire. Into the new territories, the French sent *colons*, colonists, and *bagnards*, prisoners, who had been banned from France. From the New World, they took *canne à sucre, café,* and exotic *fruits*, materials like *latex* and rubber, and *pétrole*, gas, and minerals. Some French say it was a win-win situation because they brought education, hygiene, and democracy to the New World and civilization to their subjects. The colonial *sujets*, however, may beg to differ . . .

Colonialism itself had a great influence on Dirty French. Mixed marriages, *métissage*, and hybrid cultures brought African and Asian, but mostly North African Arabic, words into the French *répertoire*. During the period of colonization, knowledge and language were regularly transferred from one side to the other. After the French were kicked out of their colonies, *les colons* came back to *la Métropole* with a different cultural and linguistic identity. Their new *vocabulaire* slowly but surely spread across the nation, reaching the important level of influence it holds today.

Finally, English has not skipped France in its worldwide domination (although France is not too pleased about this fact). Many terms, especially technical and drug related, are not Frenchified. They retain their English spellings, but are pronounced with a French accent. Examples include but are not limited to:

l'after-shave, le badge, le barbeque, le best-seller, le blue-jean, le blues, le bluff, le box-office, le break, le bridge, le bulldozer, le business, le cake, la call-girl, le cashflow, le check-in, le chewing-gum, le club, le cocktail, la cover-girl, le cover-story, le dancing, le design, le discount, le do-it-your-self, le doping, le fan, le fast-food, le feedback, le freezer, le gadget, le gangster, le gay, le hall, le handicap, le hold-up, le jogging, l'interview, le joker, le kidnapping, le kit, le knock-out, le label, le leader, le look, le manager, le marketing, le must, les news, le parking, le pickpocket, le pipeline, le planning, le playboy, le prime time, le pub, le puzzle, se relaxer, le self-service, le software, le snack, le slogan, le steak, le stress, le sweatshirt, le toaster and le week-end.

Verlan, à l'envers

Similar to the concept of English Pig Latin, *verlan* is a language made by altering French words. Unlike Pig Latin, though, *verlan* has invaded the French language at full force. Turn on the TV, flip through the newspaper, listen to a song . . . you'll hear it everywhere. *Verlan* is frequently used by *banlieuesards*, suburban youth (remember, France's suburbs are normally ghettos) and this code language has been popularized by the hip-hop scene. More than this, *verlan* is spoken by housewives, rich kids, and businessmen alike . . . they may not speak it *couramment*, but talk to them long enough and at least a few words should come out of their mouths.

Verlan transforms existing French words, including Dirty French ones, as well as foreign words into new ones by switching the syllable or reading them backward. Hence the name, *verlan* (*l'envers*, backward, becomes *verlan*, get it?). Some other transformations also occur, including shortening of the base words. This *bouquin* will provide you with some *verlan* techniques so you can understand a large part of what's to come in the next chapters.

Verlan is made in several different ways. The first example is for words with two or three syllables. The syllables are switched, placing the second syllable in first position:

> *barbu* (bar bu) becomes *bubart* (bu bar), bearded
> *arnaque* (ar nak) becomes *carna* (kar na), bad trick
> (note: the 'que' changes to a 'c')
> *celle-là* (seh la) becomes *lacelle* (la sehl), that one

Here's a list of other frequently used *verlan*:

> *fumer, méfu,* to smoke
> *merde, demèr,* shit

3

cigarette, garetci, cigarette
beau gosse, gossebo, handsome guy
famille, mifa, family
parents, rempas, parents
taper, péta, to hit
métro, tromé, underground
bizarre, zarbi, bizarre

With one-syllable words, a slightly different technique is used. Most often, you must pronounce the silent 'e' (called a schwa) at the end of the word before transforming it into *verlan*. If the word doesn't end with schwa, you must add one:

grosse (gross) becomes (gro suh) becomes *seugro* (suh gro), fat
louche (loo shuh) becomes *chelou* (shuh loo), strange
chaud (sho) becomes *auch* (oash), hot
speed (speed) becomes (spee duh) becomes *deuspi* (duh speed), fast
noir (nwar) becomes (nwah ruh) becomes *renoi* (ruh nwa), black

Shortening of the Verlan Form
As if the verlan form of a word wasn't enough, the French then cut off the end, especially if the word ends in a vowel:

SIDA becomes *dassi,* drop the 'i', becomes *dass,* AIDS
rigoler becomes *goleri,* drop the '*e*', becomes *golri,* to laugh
énervé becomes *véneré,* drop the '*é*', becomes *vénère,* angry (be sure not to pronounce the schwa)
déguisé becomes *ékisdé,* drop the '*é*', becomes *kisdé,* undercover cop

Transformation of the Base Word plus Abbreviation of the Verlan Form

Now try putting all these *verlan* tricks together to arrive at new words. First transform the word into *verlan*, then shorten it:

femme (fahm) becomes *femmeuh* (fah muh) becomes *meufa*
(muh fah) becomes *meuf* (muhf), woman, wife, or girlfriend
fête (feht) becomes (feh tuh) becomes *teufé* (tuh fay)
becomes *teuf* (tuhf), party
cher becomes (shehr) becomes (sheh ruh) becomes *reuche*
(ruh shuh) becomes *reuch* (ruhsh), expensive

Try to figure out the next progression of examples on your own:

frère—reuf, bro
mère—reum, mom
père—reup, dad
soeur—reus, sis

Re-verlanization

Sometimes words are re-verlanized, where the *verlan* word is subjected to the *verlan* process once more. For le grand final, a six-part transformation that results in the most common *verlan* word used in France today:

arabe (ah rahb) becomes (ah rah buh) becomes (buh rah ah)
becomes *beura* (buh rah) becomes *beur* (buhr), Arab

You'll hear *beur* quite often, but sometimes the process may continue:

beur (buhr) becomes *beure* (buh ruh) becomes *rebeu* (ruh
buh), Arab

Foreign Influences in French

France has quite an important gypsy, or as it is officially known Rom, population. Stereotypes abound, but *les gens du voyage*, the travelers, have an unfair reputation as criminals, beggars, and thieves. In any case, the French incorporated many Romani words into their own tongue.

gadji, f
girl, girlfriend
Cette gadji est pour moi.
That girl is for me.

gadjo, m
boy, boyfriend
Fais gaffe, ce gadjo est bizarre.
Be careful, that guy is strange.

chourer, chouraver, verlan ravchou
to steal
Ils m'ont chouré ma caisse.
They stole my car.

chouraveur, chouraveuse
thief
C'était mpossible de choper les chouraveurs.
It was impossible to catch the thieves.

chourave, f
robbery
Les gamins sont entraînés à la chourave.
Kids are trained for robbery.

chouri, surin m
knife
Il a sorti son chouri.
He took out his knife.

poucaver
to denounce, to report
Si tu poucaves, tu auras des problèmes.
If you report anything, you'll have problems.

poucaveur, poucaveuse
traitor
Les poucaveuses ont été exclues du clan.
The traitors have been banned from their clan.

maraver
to beat
J'vais te maraver grave.
I'm going to beat you hard.

bouillaver
to f**k
Je vais te bouillaver!
I'm going to f**k you!

C'est pourrave chez toi! Your house is scary (lit. your house is rotten). This is not a *Romani* word but a French one with the -*ave* suffix; *pourri*, rotten, becomes *pourrave*. This suffix is strongly associated with *les Romanichels*, the *Rom* population, especially illegal activities. As a result -*ave* makes a word sound dirtier and scarier.

Baa Baa Black Sheep

Les pieds-noirs, lit. black feet, was the name given to French colonists and settlers from North Africa, who returned to France, bringing their mixed families with them. The most famous *pied noir* was Noted Prize–winning author Albert Camus, whose works include *L'Etranger* and *La Peste*. Note the following words of Arabic origin:

barda, m
baggage, stuff
Il a pris tout son barda et est parti.
He took all his stuff and left.

bézef
a lot
Y a pas bézef dans l'assiette.
There's not a lot in the dish.

bled, m
town, village
J'viens d'un p'tit bled au Texas.
I'm from a small town in Texas.

haschich, chichon, m
hashish, lit. killer, assassin
Ils fument du chichon.
They smoke hashish.

chouia, m
a little bit, lit. small thing
J'prendrais un chouia de ça.
I'd take a little bit of that.

cador, m
dog, lit. strong, powerful
T'as sorti le cador?
Did you take the dog out?

clebs, clebard, m
dog
Fais gaffe au clebs!
Careful of the dog!

coaltar, m
daze, from the process of distillation used for black makeup
Je suis dans le coaltar—nous avons dansé et bu toute la nuit.
I'm in a daze—we were out all night dancing and drinking.

fissa
hurry, right now, lit. in the hour
Viens ici fissa!
Come here, hurry!

flouze, m
money, lit. shell
Ramène plus de flouze.
Bring more money.

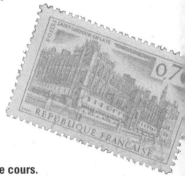

zob, m
cock
Il a sorti son zob pendant le cours.
He took out his cock during class.

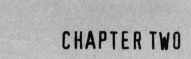

CHAPTER TWO

Laisse tomber!

Forget What Your Uptight French Teacher Taught You

We know—you either have studied French in the past or are currently attempting to master this beloved tongue. Don't let your French professor hear this, but now it's time to forget a large part of what you were taught. You must learn that people prefer it short and easy instead of long and hard. On second thought, let's save that discussion for Chapter Twenty. From now on, you've got a new set of grammar rules. Don't worry, rather than complicating things, Dirty French just simplifies them. Add these tricks to the French you've been taught and you'll miraculously start speaking like a native. Dirty French not only uses different vocabulary but is a different way of speaking altogether. So ditch the glass of wine and the beret for a cold *1664* beer and a *les Bleus* (France's national football team) cap and let these new rules flow from your tongue.

To illustrate the differences between textbook French and Dirty French, each point will be followed by an example marked **TBF** (Textbook French) and **DF** (Dirty French).

Interrogation

French has many different tools to create questions and like stinky French cheeses, not all of them are created equal. Maybe you suffered at school with the interrogative form, a Roquefort of sorts—difficult to swallow at first, but the taste grows on you. To form the interrogative, you reverse the subject and verb and put that silly little hyphen in between. Or worse, you've been less classy and used the frequent *Est-ce que* form, but still managed to sound like a foreigner.

The only way to redeem your years of sounding like an Anglophone is to phrase a question the same way you would most often in English. Speaking of English, let's call this the cheddar of questions—it doesn't look right, but it tastes damn good. Repeat the standard phrase, lifting your intonation slightly at the end of the sentence, making it 'sound' like a question. One thing that's not to be forgotten though is that every question, even when phrased like a regular sentence, needs a '?' too.

> **TBF** The inversion of the subject, *As-tu l'heure?*
> **TBF** The use of interrogative pronouns, *Qui a l'heure?*
> **TBF / DF** The use of est-ce que, *Est-ce que t'as l'heure ?*
> **DF** The tone of the voice, *T'as l'heure ?*

The two last examples are the least formal, the easiest, and as you can imagine, the most often used in Dirty French.

Omission

Omission of 'ne', the Art of Saying No

The negative form in French sounds somewhat aggressive. It's often hard to say *Je ne veux pas* or considered impolite to refuse an offer. For weak people or polite folks whose jaws struggle to say no, the elimination of the *ne* is a perfect solution. Save time by getting rid of *ne* completely and putting the emphasis on *pas*.

TBF Je n'en veux pas!
DF J'en veux pas!
I don't want any!

TBF Elle ne viendra plus chez nous.
DF Elle viendra plus chez nous.
She'll never come back to our house.

TBF Tu ne m'attires pas.
DF Tu m'attires pas.
I'm not attracted to you, lit. You don't attract me.

Omission of the 'e' in je, me, te, se, ce, que, le, petit . . .

In academic French an *e* before a vowel is never pronounced, as it's far too ugly. Imagine you've met your soul mate when you tell him or her *Comme je te aime*. Awful! Your love story may not end immediately, but your soul mate will have the impression he/she's dating a moron or a *barbare* and may regret the time they just looked into your eyes and you didn't speak a word.

The previous rule differs just a tiny bit in Dirty French. Don't pronounce the final *e* before a vowel as well as before a consonant.

TBF petit
DF p'tit
small

Sometimes, the sound is different too. The *j'* before a consonant is pronounced like the French sound for *ch* (our *sh*), as in *chat*.

TBF Je m'arrache les cheveux.
DF   J'm'arrache les cheveux.
         I'm pulling out my hair.

TBF Je rage.
DF   J'rage (pronounced shrage)
         I'm upset.

This next example is one to master immediately as actually pronouncing every word, no matter how good your French accent, will give away your tourist status every time. It's a commonly used phrase, helpful to avoid conveying your typical American 'know-it-all' attitude (at least that's how the French see you) and promote good-old Gallic indifference.

TBF Je ne sais pas.
         I don't know.
DF   Je sais pas or j'sais pas (pronounced shay pas)
         I dunno.

In the case where two words with the same initial consonant precede the elision, you may use the rule stated above, or simply hold the consonant before the elision a bit longer. When this is done correctly, you may sound like you stutter a bit—this is completely normal and means your pronunciation is quite authentic!

TBF Je te téléphone.
DF Je t' téléphone (pronounced zhuht téléphone—stutter the t's)
or
DF J' te téléphone (pronounced shtuh téléphone)
I'll call you.

Despite what you've heard about the infamous *ménage à trois*, you may never have three consonants in a row. Why not, you may ask? Just imagine pronouncing this example:

TBF Je ne te dirai rien.
DF J' t' dirai rien (hypothetically pronounced shtdirai rien)
I won't tell you anything.

You've tried, you've failed, and now you must admit that this last form is absolutely unpronounceable. So just leave your street pronunciation at the rule mentioned earlier, and pronounce these sentences accordingly:

TBF Je ne te dirai rien.
DF J'te dirai rien, pronounced shtuh dirai rien
DF Je t'dirai rien, pronounced zhuht dirai rien
I won't tell you anything.

What's the point of writing a letter you don't even pronounce? Dirty French found easy ways to gain time in both verbal and written speech. It's up to you to learn the following rules and put them to good use. Here are a few more examples to cement them in your brain:

Omission of il in il y a

TBF Il y a quelqu'un qui t'attend.
DF Y a quelqu'un qui t'attend.
There's someone waiting for you.

TBF Il y a toujours une solution.
DF Y a toujours une solution.
There's always a solution.

Omission of the re Ending

Dirty French also makes French faster and easier to write. A classic technique is to get rid of the re ending of infinitive verbs.

TBF Il n'y a rien à craindre.
DF Y a rien à craind'.
No worries, lit. There is nothing to worry about.

TBF Je ne vais pas te mordre.
DF J'vais pas t'mord'.
I don't bite, lit. I'm not going to bite you.

Omission of the u in tu

You have just learned that when placed before a word beginning with a vowel, the e of te is dropped. Well, good news for you; in Dirty French it also works with the u of tu when the word starts with a vowel.

TBF Tu attends dehors?
DF T'attends dehors?
You waiting outside?

TBF Tu envies ma réussite.
DF T'envies ma réussite.
You envy my success.

Pardon My French

It's always better to attempt more difficult French conversation, even if you're unsure of your skills. As the actress Mae West once said, "To err is human, but it feels divine." You are not a hand-held pocket translator—you are human and like all humans (yes, even the French) you will make mistakes. This is a good thing. It's important to remember that language is not static; it is constantly evolving. If not, we'd still be speaking like Shakespeare.

Whether in your mother tongue or in a foreign language, common no-no's soon become the norm. How often do you hear *ain't* when watching a reality show? Anyone with a second-grade education knows it is improper English; however, popular speech would care to disagree. Despite France's praiseworthy educational system, correct grammar, words, and verb tenses are not always used. Put some carefully chosen mistakes into your speech and you won't sound like an alien to the French.

With these errors, you may either integrate peacefully or mock French people in their own tongue (remember that American smartasses aren't much appreciated). Just be warned that the tips to come are grammatically incorrect.

Quid Pro Quo

Enseigner and *apprendre*, to teach and to learn, pose many problems for the French. Impossible to say why such a large percentage of the population makes this mistake, but fact is that they often confound learn and teach. Could it be that the French are so lazy that they expect the teacher to not only teach them, but learn for them as well?

TBF Le prof enseigne les maths aux étudiants.
The professor teaches math to the students.

DF Le prof apprend les maths aux étudiants.
The professor learns math to the students.

Incorrect Verb Tenses

Hypothetical Sentences

If you were taught textbook French, then you should already be aware that hypothetical sentences combine a hypothesis and a consequence. The hypothesis has a verb conjugated in the *imparfait de l'indicatif* or *plus-que-parfait* and the consequence takes the *conditionnel présent* or the *conditionnel passé*, respectively. If you have never heard these terms, it's time to buy a real French grammar book—the kind that elicits fear in young students—and when you've mastered the basics, pick up *Talk Dirty: French* once more.

In everyday French, you'll often hear native speakers use the *conditionnel* instead of the *imparfait*.

TBF Si tu m'aimais, tu viendrais me voir.
If you loved me, you'd come.

DF Si tu m'aimerais, tu viendrais me voir.
If you would love me, you would come.

TBF Si j'avais su, je ne serais pas venu.
If I had known, I wouldn't have come.

DF Si j'aurais su, j' serais pas venu.
If I would have known, I wouldn't have come.

This almost sounds right in English, doesn't it? No matter, it's grammatically INCORRECT!

Subjunctive Sentences

As the brightest student in your French class, you know that sentences expressing doubt, emotion, desire, or an event that has not yet happened as well as sentences with *il faut que* take the various *subjonctif* tenses. Sadly, there are four: *subjonctif présent, subjontif passé, subjonctif imparfait* and *subjonctif plus-que-parfait*. Most French people, however, limit this to the *subjonctif présent* and *subjonctif passé*.

Après que and the pronoun *que* itself are easily mixed with *avant que* or *il faut que* and cause confusion for the French novice, expert, and native alike. The use of the *subjonctif* after *que* and *après que* is blatantly wrong but extremely common.

TBF C'est le type le plus sympa que je connais.
DF C'est le type le plus sympa que je connaisse.
He's the nicest guy I know.

TBF Après que ses amies sont rentrées chez elles, Luc s'est senti tout seul.
DF Après que ses amies soient rentrées chez elles, Luc s'est senti tout seul.
After his friends left for home, Luc felt lonely.

Useless Repetitions

Dirty French likes to emphasize, exaggerate, and take pleasure in adding words that aren't necessary. Sometimes the subject of the sentence is repeated, or at other times it's the complement.

Repetition of Subject or Object

TBF Ta femme va pas bien.
 Your wife is not well.
DF Ta femme, elle va pas bien.
 lit. Your wife, she's not well.

TBF J'ai dit à ton mari de faire attention.
 I told your husband to be careful.
DF Je lui ai dit, à ton mari, de faire attention.
 lit. I told him, your husband, to be careful.

And don't think Miss Teen South Carolina is an isolated case. In France, instead of the correct form listed first, you're likely to hear the atrocious but extremely common second form:

TBF Je pense que . . .
 I think that . . .
DF Je pense personnellement que . . .
 lit. I personally believe that . . .

The French are known to be self-centered. They don't talk openly about their lives with strangers like most Americans would, but if they have something to say about themselves, they make sure the message comes across loud and clear. To put emphasis on the subject, a single 'Je' does not suffice. What's more, this double pronoun is used to draw attention to other speakers.

TBF Je ne me drogue pas.
 I don't take drugs.
DF Moi, j'me drogue pas.
 lit. Me, I don't take drugs.

TBF Qu'est ce que vous faîtes ce soir?
What are you doing tonight?

DF Vous, vous faîtes quoi ce soir?
You, you're doing what tonight?

C'est + Pronoun + qui +

Sentences with this formation should never, ever appear in written French. In Dirty French, though, they are as common as a rude waiter in Paris. When one thinks he is right, he will say *C'est moi qui a raison* rather than *J'ai raison*. In that case he may be right in his topic but from a grammatical point of view he's wrong! *C'est moi celui qui a raison* is grammatically correct but too long. You can even take this mistake to a higher level, and use the wrong verb conjugation after *qui*. For many natives, if the real subject is singular, *qui* may become its own subject, followed by the standard third person conjugation. So let the poor guy think he's right, and copy his mistake.

TBF Tu as tort or C'est toi celui qui a tort.
You're wrong.

DF C'est toi qui a tort.
lit. It's you who's wrong.

TBF J'ai dit la vérité or C'est moi celui qui a dit la vérité.
I told the truth or I'm the one who told the truth.

DF C'est moi qui a dit la vérité.
lit. It's me who told the truth.

More problems with *c'est* include using the correct conjugation when describing a plural noun. *C'est* tends to be used as the subject when in fact it should change to the plural form if the real subject is plural.

TBF/DF C'est un mensonge!
     It's a lie!
TBF Ce sont des mensonges!
     Those are lies!
DF C'est des mensonges!
     Those are lies! lit. This is lies!

Too Many Things to See

Voir (to see) is used after various commands, it seems for no particular reason other than to boss people around more politely. It has no exact translation, but can be compared to the English 'come', as in Come listen, Come watch, or Come see.

TBF Viens/écoute/touche/dis/tais-toi/regarde/attends!
     Come/listen/touch/say/shut up/watch/wait!
DF Viens voir/écoute voir/touche voir/tais-toi voir/dis voir/
     regarde voir/attends voir!
     *Come see/come listen/come touch/come shut up/come
     say/come watch/come wait!*
     *lit. Come see/listen see/touch see/shut up see/say see/
     watch see/wait see!*

The National Tendency to Exaggerate, très and trop

The French are known worldwide as overly proud and arrogant people. To listen to them, they invented democracy (what about ancient Greece?), have the most beautiful language, live in the best country in the world, and so on. This aspect of their personality is reflected in the language. Exaggeration appears in nearly every sentence. Where the usual *très* or *beaucoup* once meant a lot, really or very, now young people prefer to use *trop, grave,* or *trop grave,* which actually mean too much (lit. too serious).

TBF   Je me sens très bien dans tes bras.
        I feel really good in your arms.
DF   J'me sens trop bien dans tes bras.
        lit. I feel too good in your arms.

TBF   Je t'aime beaucoup.
        I love you a lot.
DF   J't'aime trop grave.
        lit. I love you too much.

Lexical Transformations

About the Words, Give It a Cut . . .

Dirty French can be seen as *la guillotine du langage.* Just as French revolutionaries sliced off the king's head, modern French usually slices off the end of a word . . .

TBF   maquereau, m
DF   mac, m
        pimp
        Son mac la frappe.
        Her pimp beats her.

TBF   occasion, f
DF   occase, f
        opportunity
        C'est une bonne occase pour partir.
        It's a good opportunity to leave.

TBF après-midi, m, f
DF aprèm, m, f
afternoon
On se voit pas cet aprèm.
We won't see each other this afternoon.

Or cut the beginning . . .

TBF américain, m, American
DF Ricain, m
American
Ma femme est une Ricaine.
My wife is American.

TBF musique, f, music
DF zique, f
music
Change la zique!
Change the music!

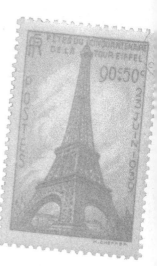

. . . *and Replace It*

Use negative suffixes to transform textbook French into more vulgar Dirty French. These suffixes all give a pejorative or comic aspect to the word, but most of the time it keeps the same meaning. The most common suffixes in Dirty French are *-ard, -asse, -iche,* and *-ot*. Those few letters give a different color to the word, which becomes rude or of lesser importance.

TBF bonne, f
DF bonniche, f
maid
Engage une bonniche!
Hire a maid!

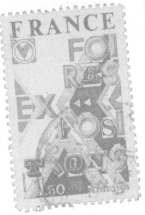

TBF con, m
DF connard, connasse
stupid, stupid bastard/bitch
Quelle espèce de connard!
What a stupid bastard!

TBF pelle, f
DF palot, m
french kiss
Roule-moi un palot.
French kiss me.

To make things look smaller just use *-et, -ette, -eau, -or, -on, -ou, -ine, -elle* . . .
This is a perfect tool to create nicknames.

TBF coquine
DF coquinelle, coquinette, coquinou
mischevous

TBF poule, f
DF poulette, f
chicken, chick
Salut les poulettes!
Hi chicks!

TBF litre, m
DF   litron, m
     liter, one-liter bottle
     Sers-nous un litron!
     Bring us a bottle of one litre!

Other suffixes are pure slang creations: *-os, -oche, -ouille,*
   -ouze, and *-lo* give a pejorative or comic aspect.

TBF gratuit
DF   gratos
     free
     L'entrée est gratos pour les meufs.
     Free entrance for women.

TBF cinéma, ciné
DF   cinoche
     movie theatre
     Allons au cinoche.
     Let's go to the movie theater.

TBF merde, f
DF   merdouille
     shit
     Merdouille, j'avais un rendez-vous y a une heure.
     Shit! I had an appointment an hour ago.

TBF piqûre, f
DF piquouse, piquouze, f
shot
Relax, c'est qu'une petite piquouse.
Relax, it's just a tiny shot.

TBF Américain, m
DF Amerlo, Amerloque, m
American
Les Amerloques envahissent Paris en été.
In summer, Americans invade Paris.

Repeating a Syllable

This easy trick is used by kids. It creates a nickname or new words in a few moves.

TBF bonne, f
DF bobonne, f
maid
J'suis pas ta bobonne.
I'm not your maid.

TBF mignon
DF mimi
cute
Comme c'est mimi.
It's so cute.

TBF fou, folle
DF foufou, fofolle
crazy
Nadia est un peu fofolle aujourd'hui.
Nadia is a bit crazy today.

Conclusion

These rules and tricks will help you create native-sounding slang words based on some 'normal' words you already possess. You'll be able to speak or understand the basics thanks to Dirty French's nifty suffixes, dropping of certain words, and shortening of other words. This chapter provides you with the skeleton, and now it's time to put some meat on those bones. Savor your new Dirty French. Delight in its emotional contents and the unexpected metaphors and poetry it contains.

NOTE: Many of the tricks explained in this chapter will be used throughout the book. Remember that your goal is not to read well, but to use Dirty French in real conversation. As a result, you will be hard pressed to find a *'ne'* written anywhere in the book, as they've already been removed to facilitate good slang pronunciation. We tried to follow the rules we just gave you.

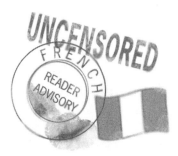

CHAPTER THREE

L'origine du monde:
Introductions and Everyday Expressions

First things first. Before you embarrass yourself entirely, let's go through what you should and shouldn't do when meeting locals. While children may give you a big hug, this won't happen with French teens and grownups. Why can't you hug the French?

People will shake hands, *se serrer la patte,* the first time they are introduced. After this initial meeting they'll usually move directly to kissing. *S'embrasser* or *se faire la bise,* to give or receive kisses on the cheeks, is the national greeting. It occurs between almost everybody, except straight guys. The only exception to shaking hands is when you are introduced to the friend of a good friend. You'll trust your friend's judgment and kiss from the get go.

It's funny that a hug is seen as an invasion of privacy, especially considering the French way of greeting people *quand la glace est rompue,* once the ice is broken—the kiss. While hugs do force direct physical contact, kisses take you right to the horse's mouth, so to speak. This *tradition* actually began in ancient Rome, when kissing was used to signify the signing of a contract. But beware of embracing this charming *coutume*, as the number of kisses can vary: two on alternating cheeks is often the rule, but you can receive up to three or four. Even the French have difficulties knowing how many times to kiss someone: social status, place of origin, and age can all play a part in this confusing game.

Another pitfall is the kissing technique. Rather than placing your lips directly on your new friend's cheeks, you must place your own cheek next to theirs, lips puckered, but making no direct contact with your lips. Ladies be warned . . . there is always a Frenchman making this little mistake on purpose to get his lips that much closer to his real target—your own.

Instead of *bonjour* and *bonsoir*, you'll hear some *salut, tchao* or *tchô*. *Tchô* was mostly used in Switzerland but was popularized in France in the 1990s thanks to the success of *Titeuf*, a breakout *suisse* comic strip. The most common greeting between close friends and family, *tchao*, is the Frenchified version of the Italian *ciao*. from *schiavo*, slave.

pépé, papi, m
grandpa, papa
Alors pépé, le viagra, ça fonctionne?
So grandpa, the Viagra, does it work?

vieux, mpl
'rents, lit. my 'olds'
Depuis qu'ils sont retraités, mes vieux s'font chier.
Since they retired, my 'rents are bored.

frérot, frangin, m
bro, from frère
Qu'est-ce qui devient ton frangin?
What's your bro up to?

'TIL DEATH DO YOU PART

If you date a French person, your *moitié* will certainly introduce you to *la belle famille*, in-laws. As brothers are usually very protective of their sisters, you will understand the meaning of the popular term *beauf*, abbreviation of *beau-frère*, brother-in-law. *Beauf* is the term for an average, closed-minded guy who spends his holidays at the same redneck resort (yes, they exist in France as well, only there they know how to choose a fine wine). *La belle-mère*, known as *la belle-maman*, lit. pretty mom, may hide her true character but *argot* will reveal it. *La belle doche*, slang for mother-in-law, indicates a nasty, harpie-like woman. Only the father and the sister-in-law don't have familiar terms, maybe because they don't have a bad reputation like *la belle-maman* and *le beauf*.

belle doche, f
mother-in-law
Les belles doches font vivre un enfer à leurs beaux-fils.
Mothers-in-law make their sons-in-law's lives into a living hell.

morveux, morveuse
kid, lit. snotty
Fais taire ton morveux ou j'lui en fous une.
Make your kid shut up or I'll slap him.

With *les rejetons*, the offspring, come a lot of slang words. While *gamin, gosse, poupon* denote good children, *morveux, mouflet, marmot, moutard, moustique* are used to describe bad kids, alluding to the filth and noise they personify.

grognasse, f
wife, girlfriend, from grogner to grumble/grunt
**Venez tous chez moi mais laissez vos grognasses à la
maison qu'on s'fasse une soirée entre mecs.**
*Everyone come to my house, but leave your girlfriends at
home so we can have a guys' night.*

Grognasse, poufiasse, pétasse, greluche, are derogatory terms for women implying stupidity. The French don't have such nasty words for friends or enemies. Friends are known as *pote, poto* or *copain,* the latter coming from the Latin *cum panis*, literally a person with whom bread is shared. Friendships tend to last longer than relationships, which may explain why Dirty French gives them much better treatment.

SO GOOD TO BE FRENCH

People of color and foreigners are described as *les métèques*. They are named after their skin color as well: *les black, les keubla (verlan), les noirs, les renoi, les jaunes,* yellow ones and *les peaux-rouge,* red skins. Some nationalities have nicknames too; *Rital* or *Macaroni* is used for

Italians, *Porto* is assigned to the Portuguese, while the Germans receive the sweet appellations of *Boches, Fritz,* and *Fridoulins. Enculé de roast-beef* covers a national food and a supposed sexual orientation and is impolitely bestowed on Brits. Americans are transformed into *Ricains, Ricaines* and *Amerloques.* During the Cold War, communists from the former USSR and Eastern Europe were called *les Coco* and *les Popovs.* Nowadays, you're more likely to hear *Russkof. Yougo* and *Youyou,* especially common in Switzerland where one full fifth of Kosovo now resides, allude to the inhabitants of the former federation of Yugoslavia.

Moving across the map, *verlan* turned *Arabes* from northern Africa into *beura, beur* and *rebeu. Raton* is also used but is extremely derogatory. The Jews are labeled *youpin;* more than sixty years after the end of WWII anti-Semitism is still present—you will still hear this word in certain areas. Asians are known as *les bridés,* the bridled ones, and *les bouffeurs de riz,* rice eaters. Chinese are known as *chinetoques* and *niakoués,* while *japs* stands for Japanese.

NOTE: These words are offensive, derogatory, and racist, and this book strongly advises that though they may penetrate your ears, they should never escape your lips.

These words are listed here because you'll hear them quite often, especially if you're traveling in the South or countryside, which was Le Pen territory in the 2002 elections. In case you've forgotten, the 2002 election featured a run-off between Jacques Chirac and the ultra-right winger Jean-Marie Le Pen. He may not have won the race, but Le Pen received a disturbing 17 percent of the vote.

Communication

faire
to go, lit. to do
Cette connasse, quand elle m'a vu, me fait: « T'as mis la robe de ta mère? »
That bitch, when she saw me, went: "Are you wearing your mom's dress?"

piger
to understand, to 'get' something
Tu piges ce que j'te dis ou bien?
Do you get what I'm saying or what?

capter
to get something, lit. to capture
J'ai rien capté là.
I didn't quite get that.

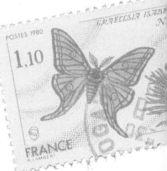

chier / chanter
to tell, lit. to shit / to sing
Qu'est-ce que tu me chies là?
What the f**k are you telling me?

radoter
to ramble, to drivel on
Chaque fois qu'Isabelle boit, elle radote.
Every time Isabelle drinks, she rambles on and on.

coller
to seem right, lit. to stick, to glue
Y a un truc qui colle pas dans ton histoire.
There's something that doesn't seem right in your story.

coincer

to hit a snag, lit. to get stuck (in something)

C'est là que ton histoire coince, le reste semblait vrai.

That's where your story hits a snag, the rest seemed true.

ne pas tourner rond

to not be quite right, lit. to turn around

Raphaël a appelé sa femme car il a senti que quelque chose ne tournait pas rond.

Raphaël called his wife because he felt something wasn't quite right.

hic, m

snag, lit. hiccup

Le hic dans tes accusations, c'est que j'étais même pas là.

The only snag with your accusations is that I wasn't even there.

blème, m

problem, abbr. of problème

Y a comme un blème.

There's a problem here.

accoucher

to tell, lit. to deliver, to give birth

Vas-y accouche!

Come on, tell!

cracher

to spit out

Crache le morceau!

Spit it out!

CHAPTER FOUR

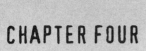

Une tête bien faite:
Smart, Stupid, and Just Plain Nuts

Knowledge and know-how should be equally divided in a *pays* that provides the same education to each one of its citizens. In a perfect world, being exposed to that *savoir* is enough to learn and retain information. But if this were the case, inner-city pupils would be at the same level as their upper middle class counterparts. As a result, severe inequalities in people's intelligence are noted. Some are brain surgeons, while others have limited capacities that leave them somewhere between George Bush and Pee Wee Herman. In a country known its criticism, the words *fraternité* and *égalité* won't stop the French from passing judgment on other people's mental capabilities.

Electricians will be pleased to note that their everyday work jargon will take them far in Dirty French—many expressions concerning mental stability and anger can be found in the electrical world. From electricity itself to cables and fuses, you'll have plenty of nasty names to call that homeless Vietnam vet or your psychotic junior-high French teacher.

Capabilities

arriver
to be able to, lit. to arrive
T'arrives à répondre à cette question?
Are you able to answer that question?

se débrouiller
to manage
J'parle pas parfaitement français mais j'me débrouille.
I don't speak French perfectly, but I manage.

se démerder
to take care, to manage, lit. to come out of the shit
J'ai pas le temps de t'aider, démerde-toi.
I've no time to help you, take care of it yourself.

avoir la bosse de qqch
to be good at something, lit. to have the bump of something
David a vraiment pas la bosse des maths.
David is really not good at math.

pointure, f
expert, lit. shoe size
**Ton Jules est une pointure en informatique; moi, j'arrive
juste à allumer un ordinateur.**
Your man is an IT expert; I can barely turn a computer on.

être un as
to be a king, lit. to be an ace
T'a réparé ma caisse? T'es un as de la mécanique.
You fixed my car? You're a mechanics king.

lumière, f

genius, lit. light

Einstein est considéré par tous comme une lumière.

Einstein is considered a genius by all.

cerveau, m

mastermind, ringleader, lit. brain

Deux semaines après l'attaque terroriste, le cerveau présumé de la bande court toujours.

Two weeks after the terrorist attack, the presumed ringleader is still on the run.

French uses words related to the brain, light, and technical terms to speak about intelligence, while female genitalia, hollow objects, and vegetables are preferred for stupidity.

stupidity

cruche, f

stupid, lit. pitcher

Maya, t'es vraiment trop cruche. Ton mec t'a quittée et t'attends encore qu'il revienne . . .

Maya, you're really too stupid. Your boyfriend left you and you're still waiting for him to come back . . .

cloche, f

moron, lit. bell

Je perds mon temps avec toi, t'es une vraie cloche!

I'm wasting my time with you, you're such a moron!

patate, f, cornichon, m

dummy, lit. potato, pickle

Alors que Béatrice donnait quelques pièces à un enfant des rues, cette patate s'est fait voler son porte-monnaie par un autre gamin.

While Béatrice was giving some change to a street urchin, that dummy got her wallet stolen by another kid!

triso, m

moron, abbr. of trisomique, a person with Down syndrome.

Tes potes se comportent parfois comme des trisos.

Your friends sometimes act like morons.

avoir de la sciure à la place du cerveau

to have shit for brains, lit. to have sawdust for brains

Réfléchis avant d'agir! C'est quoi ton problème, t'as de la sciure à la place du cerveau?

Think before reacting! What's your problem, do you have shit for brains?

crétin, crétine

cretin

Ma secrétaire est une sacrée crétine ; elle a encore oublié de poster mes lettres.

My secretary is a real cretin; she once again forgot to mail my letters.

inventer la poudre

to be clever / bright, lit. to invent powder

T'as pas inventé la poudre, toi!

You aren't so bright, are you?

ne rien avoir dans le plot / le chou

to have no brain, lit. to have nothing in the plug / in the
cabbage

**Ton mec est super mignon mais il a vraiment rien dans
le plot.**

Your boyfriend's very cute, but he has no brain.

être largué

to be incompetent, lit. to be released / abandoned

**Sophie est complètement larguée en maths. Elle a
besoin d'un coup de main.**

Sophie's completely incompetent in math. She needs help.

être paumé

to be lost, lit. to be palmed

**Hier tu voulais faire ta vie avec Lucie, aujourd'hui avec
Juliette. J'suis un peu paumé.**

*Yesterday you wanted to spend your life with Lucie, today
with Juliette. I'm a bit lost.*

Folie

perdre la boule

to go gaga, lit. to lose the ball

J'ai perdu la boule pour son accent sexy.

I went gaga over his sexy accent.

tourner la boule

to get crazy, lit. to turn the ball

**Depuis que sa femme l'a quitté pour sa meilleure amie,
Frédéric a tourné la boule.**

Since his wife left him for her best friend, Frédéric got crazy.

être marteau

to be screwy, lit. to be a hammer

Depuis son dernier accident de vélo, Daren est un peu marteau.

Since her last bike accident, Daren is a little bit screwy.

être ravagé du bocal

to be crazy, lit. to have one's jar damaged

Ivo a fait du parapente outre d'une falaise? Il est complètement ravagé du bocal ou quoi?

Ivo went paragliding off a cliff? Is he completely crazy or what?

cinglé, cinglée

lunatic (noun), insane (adjective), from cingler to hit

Jonathan conduit comme un cinglé; il a failli m'écraser avec sa voiture.

Jonathan drives like a lunatic; he nearly ran me over with his car.

dingue, dingo

nuts, crazy

Elle est dingue de toi.

She's crazy about you.

Bells are hollow, much like a stupid or crazy person's head is thought to be. When the church bells ring in France, you'll hear a ding-dong sound . . . hence the word *dingue*.

barjot, barje

crazy

Pascal est sympa et drôle, mais parfois il est vraiment barjot.

Pascal is nice and funny, but sometimes he is completely crazy.

timbré, timbrée

nuts, lit. stamped

Il faut être timbré pour penser que tous les Français sont des amants de rêve.

You've got to be nuts to think all Frenchmen are dream lovers.

manquer une case à qqn

to be missing a few blanks, lit. to miss a square

Fais pas attention à ma sœur; il lui manque une case depuis son trip au LSD.

Don't pay any attention to my sister; she's missing a few blanks since her last LSD trip.

givré, givrée

nuts, lit. frosted

Ce laideron a essayé de m'embrasser. J'suis parti— j'suis pas givré!

That ugly girl tried to kiss me. I left—I'm not nuts!

être à côté de la plaque

to be out of it, lit. to be next to the burner

Bertrand a bu que deux bières, mais il est déjà à côté de la plaque.

Bertrand has only drunk two beers, but he's already out of it.

fou / folle à lier

insane, mad, lit. crazy to bind

Lorsque Constant lui a dit qu'il allait la quitter, Camille est devenue folle à lier.

When Constant told her he was going to leave her, Camille went insane.

taré, tarée

weirdo, lit. defective

Tu dois être taré pour aller en vacances en Iraq.

You'd have to be a weirdo to go on vacation to Iraq.

maboul, maboule

weirdo, from the Arabic

Olivier a pris son antidépresseur avec un verre de whiskey. Il est maboul ou il veut finir à l'hosto?

Olivier took his antidepressant with a glass of whiskey. Is he crazy or does he want to end up in the hospital?

disjoncter

crack up, lit. to fuse

Marc a disjoncté après avoir pris trop d'héroïne.

Mark cracked up after he had taken too much heroin.

péter un câble / fusible / plomb

to go berserk, lit. to break a cable/fuse/lead

Je l'ai chicanée un peu trop et elle a pété un câble.

I teased her a little too much and she went berserk.

CHAPTER FIVE

Le roi des cons:
Words to Both Flatter and Insult

As we mentioned earlier, the French are master insulters, far ahead of other Europeans. Take their feisty Latin blood and mix with Celtic barbarian roots for a dual temperament that not only enjoys insulting others but has taken it to an art form. It is common to add insult after insult, making a long string of nasty commentary. But it's not quite as simple as you'd think . . . the key is to insult without really insulting, i.e. subtle remarks that hurt the recipient but can also be interpreted as perfectly okay if they are called into question.

These phrases are used to deliver the speaker from his or her tensions, relieving a surprising amount of anger. *Croissant* overcooked? Insult the baker. Line jumper? Make a nasty remark. Restaurant service abominable? Offend the . . . no, wait a minute, this one the French are strangely okay with. No matter how awful your waiter or waitress, complaining will give you away as a non-native every time. Your *garçon* may not seem particularly efficient, knowledgeable, or enthusiastic, but there are some bonuses to eating out in France. For one, you can stay at your table eating, talking, drinking bottle of wine after bottle of wine, and no one will push you out the door. For another, there's no tipping, as a small percentage is already included in the bill. Forget the papers and pens and pocket calculators: just leave the exact amount, perhaps rounding up to the nearest euro, and you're out the door.

Interjections

mince, zut
crap, lit. thin
Mince! J'ai encore oublié mes clefs.
Crap! I forgot my keys again.

merde
shit
**Merde! J'dois retourner au bureau pour faxer un
    contrat.**
Shit! I have to go back to work to fax a contract.

Merde can be used in every possible scenario. If you lose your keys, if you realize you forgot to do something very important, or if you're upset with someone, *merde* is your new best friend. No longer associated with the actual meaning of the word, it will barely capture the attention of the people around you when said in public, unless you're in Notre Dame for a Sunday morning service. *Merde* is also used to wish good luck before a concert premiere and in the academic world before an exam.

putain

f**k, lit. whore

Putain! Tu vois pas que j'bosse?

F**k! Can't you see I'm working?

ça fait chier / chleu

that sucks, what a bummer, lit. it makes one shit

Ça fait chier, mes vacances sont bientôt finies.

That sucks, my holiday is almost over.

bordel, m

f**k, lit. brothel

Bordel! J'ai encore perdu ma clef.

F**k! I lost my key again.

saloperie (de bordel de merde)

f**kin' a, lit. junk (from a shit brothel)

Saloperie de bordel de merde, tias-toi!

F**kin' a, shut up!

putain de bordel de merde

f**k, goddamn it, lit. whore of a shit brothel!

Fiche-moi la paix, putain de bordel de merde!

Leave me alone, goddamn it!

This is a vulgar expression whose meaning can be found in the literal translation. The term originated from an anonymous poet who frequented *une putain de bordel*, who afterward threw the contents of her *pot de chambre*, chamber pot, in his face. While best equivalents of swear words are always hard to find, the closest English translation is F**k!

Insults

To insult people there's no need to reinvent the wheel. . . . You already know a few words to describe a stupid or lazy person. In order to easily transform that knowledge into insults, easy tricks can be found by adding:

Espèce de . . .
You . . . , lit species of . . .
Espèce d'enculé!
You f**ker!

sale
dirty
Sale gamin!
Dirty kid!

sacré, sacrée
damn, lit. sacred
Sacré fils de pute!
F**king son of a bitch!

gros, grosse
fat
Grosse vache!
Fat cow!

p'tit, p'tite
small
P'tit con!
Little jerk!

Nastier Insults

enfoiré / enculé
asshole, f**khead, lit. a guy who gets f**ked in the ass
Ton chef a quitté sa femme enceinte? Quel enfoiré!
Your boss left his pregnant wife? What an asshole!

con, m
jerk, idiot, lit. cunt
Ton fils te traite de tous les mots. Quel p'tit con!
Your son calls you dirty names. What a jerk!

tête de con, m
dickhead, from con
Ton ami est un tête de con. Il m'a promis du boulot et il l'a donné à quelqu'un d'autre.
Your friend is a dickhead. He promised me a job and he gave it to somebody else.

connard, m
asshole, cunt, lit. cunt
Ton patron te dit de faire des heures sup ou il te vire? Quel connard, il n'a pas le droit!
Your boss asks you to put in extra hours or he'll fire you? What an asshole, he doesn't have the right!

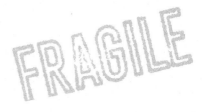

Insulting one's origin inspired *fils de pute*, son of a whore, *gosse de talus*, kid conceived on the side of the road, and *batard*.

bâtard, m
bastard
Sale bâtard! Si tu me cherches encore, j'te passe à tabac.
Dirty bastard! If you bother me again I'll kick the shit out of you.

As in English, *bâtard* has lost its primary significance and refers most often to an asshole. Remember that the French are Latin, though, and avoid putting yourself in harm's way: use it solely with those you know.

lavette, f
wimp, weak-kneed, lit. washcloth
Léo a été racketté, et cette lavette s'est pas défendue.
Léon was mugged and that wimp didn't defend himself.

femmelette / mauviette, f
wimp, lit. little woman, from mauve
Tu m'veux quoi, mauviette?
What do you want from me, wimp?

Mauviette, *femmelette*, and *lavette* refer exclusively to weak, fearful men. The use of the feminine article reinforces the derogatory aspect of the terms. These people aren't considered men at all!

chiffe molle, f

doormat, lit. soft towel

Chaque fois que je lui demande son avis, il me demande le mien. Mon mec est une chiffe molle.

Every time I ask his point of view, he asks for mine. My man is such a doormat.

petite bite, f

wimp, lit. little cock

Quelle petite bite! Il ose pas la draguer.

What a wimp! He doesn't dare flirt with her.

couille molle, f

coward, lit. soft balls

Viens ici si t'as le courage! Non? T'es vraiment qu'une couille molle!

Come over here if you have the guts! No? You're a real coward!

salaud, m

f**ker

Quelle espèce de salaud, mon père. Il a quitté le foyer lorsque j'avais deux ans.

My Dad is a real f**ker. He left home when I was only two.

râté, râtée

loser, lit. missed

Bérangère n'est qu'une ratée, elle ne fera jamais rien de bon de sa vie.

Bérangère is nothing but a loser; she won't do any good with her life.

CLOWN COLLEGE

It isn't easy to make people laugh. Few succeed, and those who don't are recognized as *bouffons*, dummies, *T'as mangé du clown au p'tit déjeuner?* (lit. Did you eat clown at breakfast?) and *T'as fait l'école du rire?*, Did you go to laugh school? Both insist on the fact that the joke or the show wasn't funny, just ridiculous. But most of the time insults bring competition between the insulter and the insulted. All weapons are permissible, as hits below the belt are standard in Dirty French.

pécno, m

country bumpkin, from *péquin*, Provençal for small

Ce pécno n'a même pas de voiture.

That country bumpkin doesn't even have a car.

fumier, m

bastard, lit. pile of manure

Ils nous interdisent de fumer à l'intérieur, les fumiers!

They ban us from smoking indoors, the bastards!

Bestiary

mufle, m

boor, lit. muffle

Quel mufle, même pas un merci!

What a boor, not even a thank-you!

chameau, m

nasty, lit. camel

Sois pas chameau avec ce mendiant.

Don't be nasty to that beggar.

porc, cochon, m
swine
Ce porc de Francis arrête pas de m'mater.
Francis, that swine, won't stop checking me out.

tête de mule, f
ass, cow (bitchy woman), lit. mule's head
J'parle plus avec cette tête de mule.
I don't talk to that cow anymore.

blaireau, m
moron, lit. badger
J'vais pas chanter pour ces blaireaux.
I won't sing for these morons.

vache, f
bastard, lit. cow
Il est vache avec toi, ton père.
Your father is a bastard to you.

huître, f
idiot, closed-minded, lit. oyster
Quelle huître!
What an idiot!

morue, f
whore, lit. cod
Quelle sale morue!
What a dirty whore!

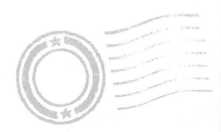

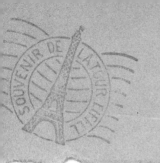

CHAPTER SIX

En route:

Time, Transportation, and Other Necessities

France is not a country of bowlers, but strikes are extremely common. Going on strike is *à la portée de tous*, everyone's right. From unhappy train conductors to miserable high school students, nearly all workers will go on strike sooner or later. Let's explore the reasons behind this uniquely French (and Italian) custom.

France has strong unions, especially in the heavy industrial sector and in the monopolistic state industries. One little strike can easily become *une grève générale*, where all workers will band together and refuse to work. Strangely, the first victims of a strike, customers, usually agree with it and give their sympathy to strikers. If you're not French and not used to *cette lutte des classes*, you'll be pissed off that the strikes usually correspond to the busiest travel times. On this note, France is not Switzerland, and trains will not depart or arrive on time. A subway ride that takes ten minutes one day can take twenty-five the next. Just changing terminals at De Gaulle airport can take an hour, and that's on a good day!

Perhaps to combat this excessive lateness, France has invested a fortune in the TGV, *train à grande vitesse*, fast train. Several of these trains now span the country, riding at speeds up to 575 kilometers or 345 miles an hour. Think the US can beat that? The fastest train in America, Amtrak's Acela, has a top speed of only 150 miles an hour!

Time

y aller mollo
to go easy, lit. to go soft
Vas-y mollo avec Nadine, elle est fragile.
Go easy with Nadine, she's vulnerable.

tout doux
slow down, lit. all smooth
Tout doux, on a plein de temps.
Slow down, we have plenty of time.

se grouiller / se magner
to hurry
Grouille-toi ou on va louper notre train.
Hurry or we'll miss our train.

avoir le feu au cul
to be in a rush, lit. to have the ass on fire
On dirait qu'il a le feu au cul.
It seems he's in a rush.

être à la bourre

to be (running) late, from an ancient French gambling card
    game, *bourre*

**Je resterais bien discuter avec toi, mais je suis à la
    bourre.**

I would gladly stay and discuss with you, but I'm running late.

être pressé

to be in a hurry, lit. to be squeezed

J'ai pas de temps pour toi, j'suis pressé.

I don't have time for you; I'm in a hurry.

être speed

to be in a hurry, lit. to be speed

J'peux pas t'aider maintenant, je suis trop speed.

I can't help you now. I'm in a hurry.

illico presto

right now

Tu le fais illico presto!

You do it right now!

plombe, f

hour, from plomb, lead

T'étais où? Ça fait une plombe que je t'attends!

Where were you? I've been waiting for you for an hour.

un jour sur deux

every other day, lit. one day on two

On se voit un jour sur deux.

We see each other every other day.

un de ces quatres

one of these days, lit. one of these fours

Nous irons boire un verre ensemble un de ces quat'.

We're going to have a drink together one of these days.

à la saint Glinglin

never, lit. on St Glinglin's day

Il a dit qu'il me paierait à la Saint Glinglin.

He told me he would never pay me back.

quand les poules auront des dents

when pigs fly, lit. when chicken have teeth

David aime la vie de célibataire. Il se mariera quand les poules auront des dents.

David loves the single life. He will get married when pigs fly.

calendes grecques, fpl

God knows when, unspecified time, from calends, a Roman division of time

Le spectacle a été renvoyé aux calendes grecques.

The show was rescheduled for God knows when.

Things

Le truc, le bidule, le machin, or *la chose* are important words that can save the day if your newfound vocabulary fails you. When you don't remember a word you can always use these generic terms interchangeably. If you have *un mot sur le bout de la langue*, a word on the tip of your tongue, *le truc* will help you save face. This expression is an extreme example for those flighty folks who just can't process too much information at the same time:

truc / bidule / machin-chose, m

stuff, thingamajig, whatchamacallit

Maria, donne-moi ce truc qui est sur le machin-chose là.

Maria, give me that thingamajig above that whatchamacallit.

bigophone, m

phone, from Bigot, French inventor

Tu m'bigophones ce soir, d'accord?

You'll call me tonight, okay?

coup de fil, m

phone call, lit. hit of thread

J'attends toujours son coup de fil . . .

I'm still waiting for his phone call . . .

lourde, f

door, lit. heavy

Ferme la lourde, s.t.p.!

Close the door, please!

bouquin, m

book

Elle a acheté pour cent euro de bouquins.

She bought one hundred euros worth of books.

canard, m

newspaper, lit.a duck

**Des photos du président saoul sont dans tous les
canards.**

Pictures of the drunken president are in every newspaper.

papelard, m

paper, documents, file

La secrétaire trouve plus le papelard qu'elle doit envoyer au plus vite.

The secretary can't find the file she has to send as soon as possible.

toc, m

fake

Il est pas en or ton collier ; c'est du toc!

Your collar isn't made of gold; it's fake.

toquante, f

watch

Paul a foutu en l'air sa toquante en nageant dans la mer.

Paul ruined his watch by swimming in the sea.

Cars

In a country of individualism, the most important object is the one that provides you with freedom. As the Germans had their Volkswagen, French had their Citroën. The model equivalent to the VW Bug or Beetle was *la deuch, la deux chevaux*, the two horsepower. French authorities nationalized the most important car factories, those of Peugeot and Citroën. As a product beloved by the masses, the car developed massive slang terms as well.

aimant à femmes, m

chick magnet, lit. women magnet

Ma Porsche, c'est un vrai aimant à femmes.

My Porsche is a total chick magnet.

bétaillère, f

slow car, lit. bull-hauler

Tu vas bouger ta bétaillère ou je dois venir la déplacer?

Are you going to move your slow car or do I have to do it?

veau, m

boat (big car), lit. veal

Tu m'fais pas conduire ce veau; louons une cabriolet.

You can't make me drive this boat; let's rent a convertible.

tacot / clou, m

jalopy, lit. crate / nail

Le tacot de ton mec fait tache.

Your boyfriend's jalopy is an eyesore.

lit. Your boyfriend's nail makes a stain.

tape-cul, m

shitty car, lit. car that hits the ass

T'arrives pas à faire monter Alyssa dans ton tape-cul.

Alyssa won't take a ride in your shitty car.

bolide, m

hot rod, lit. projectile

Mon voisin s'est acheté un bolide de marque.

My neighbor bought himself a hot rod.

bleu, m

driver's license, lit. blue

**Le policier a retiré le bleu de Joy, car cette folle de
biffteck roulait du mauvais côté de la route.**

*The policeman took Joy's license away because that crazy Brit
was driving on the wrong side of the road.*

virée, f

spin, joyride, from virer, to heave

Ma copine veut faire une virée en voiture ce week-end.

My girlfriend wants to take the car out for a spin this weekend.

faire péter le compteur

to drive fast, lit. to make the speedometer explode

Vas-y Alain, fais péter le compteur!

Go on, Alain, drive fast!

pied au plancher

pedal to the metal, lit. foot to the wooden floor

Pour un beau dérapage, mets le pied au plancher et tourne le volant.

For a nice skid, put the pedal to the metal and turn the steering wheel.

planter les gommes

to brake, lit. to plant the gums

Le conducteur a planté les gommes au dernier moment.

The driver braked at the last second.

recevoir une bûche

to get a ticket, lit. to get a log

Lucien a reçu une bûche car il a parqué sur une place pour handicapés.

Lucien got a ticket because he parked in a space reserved for disabled people.

lever le pied

to slow down, lit. to lift the foot

Simon a vu la bagnole de flic cachée derrière l'arbre et a levé le pied immédiatement.

Simon saw the police car hidden behind the tree and slowed down immediately.

brûler un stop / un feu rouge

to run a red light, lit. to burn a stop / a red traffic light

Mikkel a brûlé un stop et a été pincé par un flic.

Mikkel ran a red light and got caught by a policeman.

bouchon, m

traffic jam, lit. cork

Nous sommes bloqués dans un bouchon.

We're blocked in a traffic jam.

CHAPTER SEVEN

À table:
Food, Glorious Food

Ask anyone where the best food in the world comes from and their answer will undoubtedly be France. Good cooking may run in their blood, but maintaining this status is hard work. The finest food often requires awful treatment of *la matière première*, the source. The process of making *foie gras*, for example, is now considered abuse and illegal in many places in the US and UK. Except for a handful of PETA devotees, if you asked the French if *foie gras* was cruel they'd laugh in your face. Other French favorites include *les cuisses de grenouille*, frog's legs, and *les escargots à l'ail*, snails in garlic butter. As the French say, *il faut goûter de tout*, one must taste everything, loosely rendered as "Don't knock it 'til you've tried it." *La tête de veau vinaigrette*, calf's head in vinegar dressing, is one of the preferred meals of the former President Jacques Chirac. And you thought Clinton's McDonald fetish was weird!

table, f
restaurant, lit. table
Tu connais une bonne table dans le coin?
Do you know a good restaurant in the area?

resto, m

restaurant, abbreviation of restaurant

**On peut se faire un chinois, un italien, ou un indien . . .
ce sont pas les restos qui manquent près d'ici.**

*We can do Chinese, Italian, or Indian . . . there's no lack of
restaurants around here.*

grailler

to eat

Y a jamais rien à grailler dans notre frigo!

There's never anything to eat in our fridge!

crever de faim

to die of hunger

**Il faut que ta copine graille quelque chose. Regarde-la,
elle crève de faim !**

*Your friend needs to eat something. Look at her, she's dying of
hunger!*

avoir la dalle / fringale

to be hungry, lit. to have the pavement stone

Quand Madeleine a la dalle elle devient méchante.

When Madeleine is hungry she gets mean.

avoir les crocs

to be hungry, lit. to have fangs

T'as rien cuisiné et j'ai les crocs.

You haven't cooked anything and I'm hungry.

manger un morceau / une petite morse

to grab a bite, lit. to eat a piece/mouthful

Si t'as faim, on peut aller se manger une petite morse.

If you're hungry we can grab a bite to eat.

grignoter qqch

to snack/nosh on something

C'est fou! Il faut toujours que tu grignotes quelque chose au cinéma.

It's crazy! You always have to nosh on something at the movie theater.

casse-croûte, m

snack, lit. crust breaker

Mon casse-croûte préféré est un panini.

My favorite snack is a panini.

gueuleton, m

feast, from gueule (mouth, for animals)

On se fait un gueuleton entre copines?

Should we have a ladies' night feast?

bouffer

to eat (for animals)

Tais-toi et bouffe!

Shut up and eat!

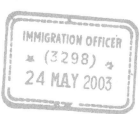

à gogo

all you can eat

Chaque samedi soir, la pizzeria à côté propose des pizzas à gogo.

Every Saturday, the pizzeria next door has all you can eat pizza.

se taper l'incruste

to invite oneself, lit. to hit oneself the incrusted

Marvin s'est encore une fois tapé l'incruste pour dîner.

Marvin invited himself over again for dinner.

fine-gueule, f

gourmet, lit. thin mouth

Les fines-gueules évitent les buffets.

Gourmets avoid buffets.

cuistot, m

cook, from cuisinier

Bethany est un bon cuistot.

Bethany is a good cook.

malbouffe, f

junk food, lit. bad food

La malbouffe envahit l'Europe.

Bad food is invading Europe.

Food is still a passion and a vital part of French culture, but fast food is slowly creeping into the French lifestyle. *Les Français* are also losing their two-hour lunch break as women work more and more, depriving them of the time to cook. The result? Not only are families spending less time together, but obesity cases are quickly on the rise. Not to worry, though, the French paradox—a diet of cheese, creamy sauces, copious amounts of red wine and a stunningly slim figure—still holds true in most areas. It's also interesting to see that this new way of eating is inspiring the creation of slang. Have you heard about *un mc job*?

avoir un bon coup de fourchette
to eat a lot, lit. to have a good hit with a fork
Il est maigre mais il a un bon coup de fourchette.
He's very slim but he really eats a lot.

se goinfrer
to stuff oneself
Arrêtez de vous goinfrer de friandises.
Stop stuffing yourselves with sweets.

bâfrer
to eat like a pig, lit. to eat greedily
Elles se sont bâfrées et sont parties sans payer.
They ate like pigs and left without paying the bill.

bidoche / barbaque, f
meat, from a French *patois* word meaning old sheep
J'ai envie de bouffer de la bidoche.
I feel like eating meat.

poiscaille, m
fish, from poisson
Y a du poiscaille à midi.
There's fish for lunch.

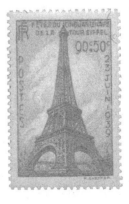

from', m / frometon, m
cheese, abbr. of fromage
Oublie pas le frometon!
Don't forget the cheese!

CHAPTER EIGHT

Les fleurs du mal:
Beer Before Liquor . . .

Drinking alcohol is an integral part of French culture. It is quite normal to drink *vin* every day, and even the kids are allowed to have some wine diluted with water. France is a predominantly Catholic country and after all—if wine is the blood of their savior, then to drink it at every meal should be considered an act of faith.

Ask anyone (ok, maybe not a Californian) where the best *vin* in the world is produced and you'll hear the same answer time after time: France. No longer is French wine a treat for the wealthy though; bottles of *Beaujolais nouveau* now abound at every 7-11. As wine sales increase in the United States, the opposite is happening in France. Since 2000, wine exports have dropped 6 percent and the country has lost more than one million wine drinkers—and it's not because they died of cirrhosis. Persuasive health campaigns are mostly to blame for alcohol's rapid decline. Old-school French mourn the loss of daily wine-soaked lunches, and can't bear the thought of bière becoming the most popular beverage for Generations X and Y.

But in case you doubt America's role in winemaking, read on. Did you know that all European wines, even French wines, are distinctly American? In 1860, a British scientist took *vignes* from the US back to England for study. From these vines, the bug *Phylloxera* spread over the Continent, destroying nearly all the vineyards in Europe. There was no other solution than to import vines from the New World, which were naturally resistant to the bug. European grape varieties were then grafted onto the American vines to retain the distinct species. So except in a few very rare cases, there are no more proper European vines . . . while the grapes may be French, the roots are American!

crever de soif
to die of thirst
Je crève de soif. Fais péter une bouteille de chardonnay.
I'm dying of thirst. Pop open a bottle of chardonnay.

aller boire un coup
to go for a drink, lit. to go drink a knock
Allons boire un coup—j'offre la première tournée.
Let's go for a drink—the first round's my treat.

partir en piste
to go out for a drink, lit. to go on a trail
Qu'est-ce qui se passe? C'est samedi soir et t'as pas envie de partir en piste.
What's wrong? It's Saturday night and you don't want to go out for a drink.

bistro, bistrot, m
bar, café
On va prendre un verre au bistrot du coin.
We are going to have a drink at the café on the corner.

tord-boyaux, m
(bad) booze, lit. that bends the guts
Jette-moi loin cette merde de tord-boyaux!
Throw away this shitty booze!

tournée, f
round (of drinks), lit. turn
Patron, j'offre la tournée générale!
Boss, a round for the house on me!

mousse, f
beer, lit. foam
Mademoiselle, vous nous remettez trois mousses?
Miss, can you bring us three beers?

bibine, f
beer
On fait quoi, Bruno? On reprend une bibine?
What are we doing, Bruno? Are we having another beer?

pinard, m
wine, lit. bad wine
Je vous ai amené une bouteille de pinard fait par mes vieux.
I brought you a bottle of wine made by my parents.

vinasse, f
lousy wine
Beurk! Quelle vinasse, même pas bonne pour un coq au vin!
Yuck! What lousy wine, not even good enough for a coq-au-vin!

A MATTER OF SIZE

Beer, like wine, is serious business in France as well as the rest of Europe. No matter the kind of beer, customers will order the brand they love in the glass they prefer. For light drinkers or ladies, *un galopin* or *un bock* (0,125L) will suffice. A thirstier client will ask for *une demi chope* or *un demi*, the abbreviation of *demi-pinte*, half a pint (0,25L). During *les canicules*, heatwaves, the customers will rebuild their bodies' water reserves with *une chope*, a mug. Other classic beer glasses with a handle include *un baron, une pinte, un sérieux,* or *un mini chevalier* (0,50L). *Une double pinte, un parfait, un formidable, un chevalier,* are the drunkards' favorites. It's not only cheaper to buy per liter but more ecological as well. Here's a message for Al Gore: Save the planet, drink more beer!

cul-sec
bottoms up, lit. ass-dry
Finis ton verre cul-sec ou on va louper le début du film.
Bottoms up! Finish your drink or we'll miss the beginning of the movie.

arrosé, arrosée
swimming in alcohol, lit. watered
La soirée est bien arrosée.
The party is swimming in alcohol.

se déchirer
to get plastered, lit. to tear oneself
Mon cousin s'est déchiré à l'absinthe.
My cousin got plastered on absinthe.

se péter le tube

to get drunk, to get loaded, lit. to break the tube

Après le repas, les femmes ont discuté entre elles tandis que les maris se pétaient le tube au bourbon.

After the meal, the women discussed amongst themselves while the husbands got loaded on bourbon.

fin caisse

drunk, trashed, lit. end of the (wine) case

Marion était fin caisse après ses deux verres de whiskey. J'ai dû la porter à la maison.

Marion was trashed after two glasses of whiskey. I had to carry her back home.

se prendre une torchée

to get drunk, lit. to take a wipe

Depuis qu'il s'est pris une torchée au pastis, Thomas ne supporte plus le goût d'anis.

Since he got drunk on pastis, Thomas can't stand the flavor of anise any more.

se biturer, se prendre une biture

to get wasted, lit. to drink oneself, from béture, boisson, drink

Pour fêter, j'ai décidé de me prendre une biture.

To celebrate, I've decided to get wasted.

se saouler (la gueule)

to get drunk

Ça fait une paye que nous nous sommes plus saoulés la gueule.

It has been a long time since we have gotten drunk.

pomper

to drink, lit. to pump

T'as de l'aspirine? J'ai trop pompé à la fête de Stéphanie et j'ai mal au caillou.

You got some aspirin? I drank too much at Stéphanie's party and my head hurts.

être pompette

to be slightly drunk, from pomper

Petite précision: je ne suis pas complètement saoul. Je suis seulement un peu pompette.

Correction: I'm not completely drunk. I'm only buzzed!

lever le coude

to drink, lit. to lift the elbow

Gaétan a trop levé le coude—il est malade depuis deux jours.

Gaétan drank too much—he's been sick for two days.

tiser

to drink

Yves et Déborah ont tisé toute la nuit à la fête de Marie-Laure. Aucun des deux n'a pu conduire pour rentrer, alors ils ont dormi chez elle!

Yves and Déborah drank all night at Marie-Laure's party. Neither one of them could drive home, so they slept at her place.

se cuiter, prendre une cuite

to get drunk, lit. to get cooked

Les jeunes se cuitent le week-end en groupe.

Young people get drunk in groups on the weekend.

ivre-mort

dead drunk

C'est assez rare en Europe de voir une femme ivre-morte.

It's pretty rare in Europe to see a woman dead drunk.

Conséquences

alcoolo, m, f

alcoholic, short for alcoolique

Vivre avec un alcoolo demande beaucoup de patience.

Living with an alcoholic requires a lot of patience.

éponge, f

sponge

Il a bu cinq litres de vin? Ton ami est une éponge!

He drank five liters of wine? Your friend is a sponge!

ivrogne, m, f

drunkard, from ivre, drunk

Arrête de te plaindre l'ivrogne! On aimerait avoir la paix!

Stop complaining, you drunkard! We'd like some peace and quiet!

pilier de bar, m

regular, lit. bar pillar

Une prostituée est devenue un pilier du bar de notre quartier.

A prostitute has become a regular at our neighborhood bar.

souillard, souillasse

wino, derogatory term of soûl, drunken

Cette souillasse d'Elaine est pas encore rentrée.

That wino Elaine hasn't come back yet.

dégueuler / dégobiller

to throw up, from gueule / gola, mouth

C'est pas rigolo de dégueuler des spaghettis!

It's not funny to throw up spaghetti!

déballer

to throw up, lit. to unwrap

Bénédicte a tout déballé dans le lavabo de la salle de bain.

Bénédicte threw up everything in the bathroom sink.

French youth follow the mantra *Blanc sur rouge, rien ne bouge—Rouge sur blanc, tout fout le camp*, literally, "White on red" (referring to the levels of wine sitting atop one another in the stomach) "[,] nothing moves—Red on white, everything goes away" (you will throw everything up). Much like the US youth who say, "Beer before liquor, you've never been sicker—Liquor before beer, you're in the clear," or that you should start with strong alcoholic drinks and finish with light ones and never the opposite. The French, however, believe exactly the opposite. When asked, they'll tell you to start with a light alcoholic drink and finish up with a strong one!

être dans le coaltar

to be in a daze, to be out of it, lit. to be in the asphalt

Je suis encore dans le coaltar et j'comprends pas c'que tu m'dis.

I am still out of it and can't understand what you're telling me.

avoir la tête dans le cul

to have a hangover, lit. to have the head in the ass

Les noceurs se sont réveillés avec la tête dans le cul.

The partiers woke up with a hangover.

gueule de bois, f

hangover, lit. wooden face

Après le mariage, les invités avaient tous la gueule de bois.

After the wedding, the guests all had hangovers.

bouche pâteuse, f

cotton mouth, lit. doughy tongue

T'as pas un verre d'eau? J'ai la bouche toute pâteuse de hier soir.

You don't have a glass of water? I have cotton mouth from last night.

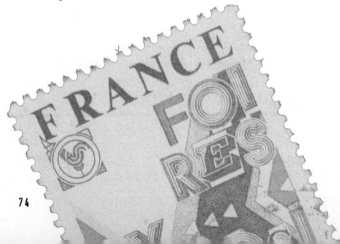

CHAPTER NINE

Joie de vivre:

Expressing Your Ups and Downs

French *classicisme* proved one of the most influential movements in history. Great writers and playwrights such as Jean Racine and Pierre Corneille used ancient Roman and Greek 'rules' to push formal and restrained principles in literature. From here, French classicism spread into all areas of life. But France today is not only a country of reason, knowledge, and high virtues—*émotions* are very present in daily life. If courage is the secret garden of classicism, then fear, anger, and envy, are the privileged *domaine* of Dirty French.

Except for a short period, during German occupation and under the Vichy government, freedom of *expression* has been catapulted to a very high level in France. The truth-talking and truth-mocking tone in France is impossible to duplicate in other countries. Political *journaux* and shows on TV are given a completely different image than the one desired by the communication counselors of the successive governments. Journalists from *Le canard enchaîné* or imitators from *Les guignols de l'info* (a puppet-led phony news program), as well as some comics, take great pleasure in telling the truth or causing governments to fall. *Toutes les vérités sont bonnes à dire,* all truths are good to tell, and humor is still the best way to share a point of view. The information given by the media has great influence on the French, who are always unhappy with their government and eager to believe a TV program over their President.

Intérêts et désintérêts

en jeter / mettre plein la vue
to show off, lit. to throw / put into view
Pascal roule en Mercedes pour en mettre plein la vue.
Pascal drives a Mercedes to show off.

géant, grandiose
great, lit. giant, grandiose
C'est géant—je l'ai battu douze fois de suite au babyfoot!
It's great—I beat him twelve times in a row at foosball!

être emballé par qqch
to be thrilled, lit. to be wrapped up
J'suis pas trop emballé par ton idée!
I'm not so thrilled by your idea!

cartonner
to do really well
La nouvelle chanson d'U2 cartonne au top 50!
U2's new song has already made the Top 50!
Or
to blow something
Cet examen, ne m'en parle plus—j'ai cartonné.
Don't talk to me about this test anymore—I blew it.

faire un tabac

to be a great success. lit. to make a tobacco

Le dernier film de Depardieu a fait un tabac.

Depardieu's last movie was a great success.

s'arracher

to snatch up, lit. to tear off, pull out

Chaque quat' ans, les gosses s'arrachent les vignettes du mondial de foot.

Every four years, kids snatch up stickers of the soccer world championship.

crever d'envie

to be dying to, lit. to die of want

Je crève d'envie de quitter mon boulot!

I am dying to quit my job!

crever de jalousie

to die of envy

Daliha est allée à Cannes pour le festival—et sa meilleure amie en crève de jalousie.

Daliha went to Cannes for the festival—and her best friend is dying of envy.

botter

to dig something, lit. to kick (with a boot)

Ça me botte, votre idée de voyager en autostop.

I dig your idea of a hitchhiking trip.

bof

uh, um

Tu as envie d'aller à la piscine? Bof, pas vraiment.

Do you want to go to the pool? Um, not really.

en avoir rien à cirer / à battre

to not give a damn, lit. to have nothing to wax/beat

Le premier ministre en a rien à cirer des chômeurs.

*The prime minister doesn't give a damn about the
    unemployed.*

en avoir rien à branler / à foutre

to not give a shit, lit. to have nothing to wank about/to do (f**k)

Ta miss t'a quitté? J'en ai rien à branler!

Your girlfriend left you? I don't give a shit!

s'en battre les couilles / l'œil

to not give a shit, lit. to beat one's balls / one's eye

Je m'en bats les couilles de tes histoires de cul.

I don't give a shit about your sex stories.

nul à chier

awful, f**king bad, lit. so bad that it makes someone shit

T'as aimé le dernier Lelouche? Non, il était nul à chier.

Did you like the last Lelouche film? No, it was so f**king bad.

merde, f

piece of crap, shit

C'est de la merde!

That's a piece of crap!

navet, m

rotten tomato, lit. turnip

**J'aime bien Gérard Jugnot, mais il a joué dans pas mal
    de navets dans sa carrière.**

*I really like Gérard Jugnot, but he's played in quite a few rot-
    ten tomatoes in his career.*

bijou, m

jewel

Le bouquin que tu lis est un petit bijou.

The book you're reading is a real jewel.

Colored Emotions

être vert / verte de jalousie

to be green with envy

Mon collègue a reçu une promotion et je suis vert de jalousie.

My co-worker got a promotion and I am green with envy.

être rouge de rage

to be red with anger

Quand ma mère a surpris mon père au lit avec une autre femme, elle était rouge de rage.

When my mother surprised my father in bed with another woman, she was red with anger.

broyer du noir

to be down in the dumps, lit. to grind black

Depuis que mon oncle est mort, je broie du noir.

Since my uncle died I've been down in the dumps.

avoir des idées noires

to have dark thoughts, lit. to have black ideas

Arrête d'avoir des idées noires et regarde le bon coté des choses.

Stop having dark thoughts and look on the bright side!

Fear Factor

chair de poule, f
goose bumps, lit. chicken flesh
Lorsqu'Emma me touche, j'ai la chair de poule.
When Emma touches me, I get goose bumps.

craignos
scary
Vivre en banlieue parisienne, c'est craignos!
To live in the Paris suburbs is scary.

foutre les jetons à qqn
to scare somebody stiff, lit. to throw down the chips to someone
Ne me fais plus jamais ça! Tu m'as foutu les jetons!
Don't ever do that to me again. You really scared me!

avoir les chocottes
to be scared stiff, lit. to have teeth that chatter
**A l'approche des examens, les mauvais étudiants ont
    les chocottes.**
As exams approach, bad students are scared stiff.

avoir la trouille
to be scared shitless, lit. to fear
**Arrête de te la jouer! Tout le monde peut voir que t'as la
    trouille.**
Stop trying to act cocky! Everyone can see you're scared shitless.

foutre la frousse à qqn
to scare the living daylights out of someone
La situation du Proche-Orient me fout la frousse.
The Middle East situation scares the living daylights out of me.

So French

ne plus se sentir pisser

to be walking on air, lit. to not feel oneself pee

Luc ne se sent plus pisser depuis que la chaudasse de l'hôtel lui a donné son numéro de chambre . . .

Luc has been walking on air since the hottie at the hotel gave him her room number . . .

se la péter / jouer

to act cocky, lit. to explode / to play

Momo se la joue trop depuis qu'il a acheté une nouvelle tire!

Momo acts so cocky since he bought a new car!

pousser un coup de gueule / une gueulée

to let out a yell, lit. to push a hit of the mouth

Pour rétablir l'ordre dans son auditoire, le prof a poussé une gueulée.

In order to restore quiet in his auditorium, the professor let out a yell.

tirer la gueule

to be in a huff, lit. to pull the mug

J'aimerais savoir pourquoi tu tires la gueule.

I'd like to know why you're in such a huff.

avoir les boules

to be / to get upset, lit. to have balls

Yannick a les boules quand il voit comment le copain de sa sœur la traite.

Yannick gets upset when he sees how his sister's boyfriend treats her.

tiquer

to wince, lit. to tick

Edgar a tiqué quand tu t'es moqué de lui.

Edgar winced when you made fun of him.

faire le grognon

to grumble

Pourquoi tu fais le grognon?

What are you grumbling about?

bouder

to sulk

Ne reste pas là à bouder dans ton coin, viens avec nous!

Don't sit in your corner and sulk, come with us!

grincheux, m

grouch

**Le grincheux qui habite en dessous de moi me rend la
  vie impossible.**

The grouch that lives below me makes my life impossible.

être bougon

to be grumpy

Chris est tout bougon depuis que Lisa l'a quitté.

Chris has been grumpy since Lisa left him.

être mal luné

to be in a bad mood, lit. to be badly 'mooned'

**Nous ne faisons plus de cas de Stéphanie. Ça fait une
  semaine qu'elle est mal lunée.**

*We don't pay attention to Stéphanie anymore. She has been
  in a bad mood for a week.*

faire une boulette

to make a little mistake, lit. to make a little ball

Oups, je crois que j'ai fait une boulette.

Oops, I think I made a little mistake.

péter plus haut que son cul

to think one's shit doesn't stink, lit. to fart higher than one's
     ass

Jacques pète plus haut que son cul ou quoi?

Jacques thinks his shit doesn't stink or what?

avoir qqch dans la peau

to have something in one's blood, lit. to have something in the
     skin

Kristine a le rythme dans la peau.

Kristine has rhythm in her blood.

Jokes

blaguer

to talk, to joke

Nous avons blagué avec nos amis jusqu'au petit matin.

We talked with our friends until early in the morning.

blague, f

joke

C'est vraiment une mauvaise blague.

That's really a bad joke.

rigoler

to joke around from *rire*, to laugh

On a rigolé tout l'après-midi.

We joked around all afternoon.

se marrer

to have a lot of fun

On ne se marre pas tous les jours.

We don't always have a lot of fun.

se fendre la gueule / se poiler

to laugh hysterically, lit. to split one's face / to 'hair' oneself

Le public s'est fendu la gueule en écoutant le discours débile du speaker.

The audience laughed hysterically while listening to the speaker's stupid speech.

raconter des bobards / des salades

to tell lies, lit. to tell bobbins/salads

C'est pas des bobards, crois-moi.

They aren't lies, believe me.

se foutre / ficher de la gueule de qqn

to make fun of someone, lit. to do someone's face

Tu te fiches de ma gueule ?

Are you making fun of me?

gober

to buy, lit. to swallow, from gola, mouth

T'as gobé son histoire ?

Did you buy her story?

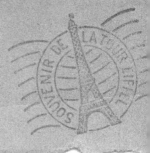

CHAPTER TEN

Rien qu'une brique dans le mur:
Yes, You Do Need an Education

French *argot* was not invented by aristocrats, nobility, or other wealthy, educated people. Slang was, and is today, most influenced by the lower classes. Poverty, unemployment, and people of the streets—prostitutes, bums, workers, and artisans—provide the biggest contribution to the evolution of *français*. Real life in general, far away from Versailles and its parties, the church, or nobility, is the main source of slang *vocabulaire* and unusual phrases.

With masters like Blaise Pascal and René Descartes, France has a long history of scientific success. They used this talent for crunching numbers in many ways, from Pascal's famous *triangle* to the invention of the 35-hour workweek. They figured by reducing working hours from 39 to 35, those four hours would, when combined, add up to many new jobs. In a mathematically perfect world, this equation would have worked. French *employeurs*, however, didn't see things quite the same way. Now, workers are forced to finish the same tasks they once did in 39 hours in only 35 hours, for four hours less pay! And as you can see below, the number of slang expressions for laziness means that employers think they can do even better.

Workplace

bahut, m

high school, lit. sideboard, hutch

Simon attend tous les jours Renée devant la porte du bahut.

Simon waits for Renée at the high school entrance every day.

bachot, m

baccalaureate

Il a son bachot dans la poche.

He has his high school diploma in the pocket.

poser une colle

to ask a tricky question, lit. to put a glue

Là, tu me poses une colle et j'sais pas la réponse.

You're asking me a tricky question, and I don't know the answer.

être collé

to have a school detention, lit. to be glued

J'me suis jamais fait collé en classe.

I've never had detention.

sécher

to not know the answer, lit. to dry

J'ai complètement séché sur la question lors de l'oral.

I didn't know the answer to the question at the oral exam.

antisèche, f

cheat sheet, lit. anti-dry

Avec ses antisèches, Alain réussit tous les tests.

With his cheat sheets, Alain passes every test.

bizut, m

newcomer, from bizuter, to bully, to haze

Je déteste comme les confréries d'étudiants traitent les bizuts.

I hate how fraternities treat their newcomers.

bizutage, m

hazing, from bizuter

Les bizutages sont dangereux et stupides.

Hazing is dangerous and stupid.

taf, m

job, from Arabic

Tous les matins, faut se lever pour aller au taf.

Every morning, you've got to get up to go to work.

boulot, m

work, from boule, ball

Tous les jours c'est le même refrain: métro, boulot, dodo.

Every day it's the same old story: eat, work, sleep.

lit. Every day it's the same old chorus: subway, work, sleep.

usine, f

work, office, lit. factory

Merde, c'est déjà l'heure de retourner à l'usine.

Shit, it's time to go back to work already.

travailler au noir
to work under the table, lit. to work in the black
Dorothée travaille au noir dans un salon de coiffure.
Dorothée works illegally in a hair salon.

virer qqn
to fire somebody
Le patron a viré son mauvais vendeur.
The boss fired his poor salesman.

Professions and Social Status

aristo, m, f
aristocrat, abbr. of aristocrate
Y a encore quelques aristos en France.
There are still some aristocrats in France.

clochard, clocharde, charclo in verlan / clodo, m, f
bum, from cloche, bell
Les clochards dorment dans des cartons dans les rues.
Bums sleep in cardboard boxes on the streets.

What connects a bum and a bell? Historically, bums survived thanks to the charity of the church and the leftovers given to them. What better way to call these people to eat than using a small bell? Bums were in a certain way surviving only thanks to the bell, *cloche;* hence they became *clochards.* Nowadays the appellation *SDF,* abbr. of *Sans Domicile Fixe,* homeless, is the preferred term.

prolo, m
proletarian, abbr. of prolétarien
Y a de plus en plus de prolos qui votent à droite.
There are more and more proletarians that vote for the right.

instit, m, f
teacher
Mon nouvel instit est trop cool.
My new teacher is too cool.

bobo, m, f
bobo, abbr. of bourgeois Bohême
Devenir bobo est une mode.
To become a bobo is a trend.

baba cool, m, f
hippie
Ma mère s'fringue toujours en baba cool.
My mom still dresses like a hippie.

bourge, m, f
middle class citizen, abbr. of bourgeois
T'es qu'un sale bourge.
You're nothing but middle class.

Conchita de service, f
maid, lit. maid named Conchita
**Ramasse tes affaires et range ta chambre. J'suis pas la
    Conchita de services.**
Pick up your things and clean your room. I'm not the maid.

bonniche, f

maid, from bonne, maid

Les bonniches connaissent tous les secrets des femmes et couchent parfois avec les maris.

Maids know all the wives' secrets and sometimes sleep with the husbands.

larbin, m

groom, slave, lit. valet

J'suis pas ton larbin alors tu me causes autrement.

I'm not your slave so you'd better speak to me differently.

cul-terreux, m

hillbillies, lit. muddy ass

Chaque samedi, les culs-terreux viennent vendre leurs légumes au marché.

Every Saturday, the hillbillies come to sell their vegetables at the market.

politicard, m

politician, from politician

Les discours des politicards ne sont que de belles paroles.

Politicians' speeches are nothing but sweet words.

bidasse, f

soldier

Les bidasses se saoulent souvent pendant leurs sorties.

Soldiers often get drunk when they go out.

bleusaille, f

rookie, from bleu, blue, color of the recruit's uniform

Elle me veut quoi la bleusaille?

What does the rookie want from me?

Every group creates its own rules, traditions, and slang, and the army is no different. Blue was the color of the uniform of military recruits and is now synonymous with an inexperienced person in any field.

bosser

to work, lit. to make a hump

Nous avons bossé comme des esclaves toute l'année. Nos vacances sont plus que méritées.

We worked like slaves all year long. Our vacation is more than deserved.

The *bosse* family is connected with work. The concept of working so hard it physically deforms you can be found in *se courber sur le travail, se plier à la tâche,* to bend on the work, or the really vulgar *se casser le cul au travail,* to break one's ass at work. Keep this in mind when someone tells you that work is healthy and leisure unhealthy. Unlike most overachieving Americans, the French believe that one shouldn't mistreat his body. After all, *le travail c'est la santé—rien faire c'est la conserver.*

rouler sa bosse

to knock about, to travel aimlessly, lit. to roll one's hump

J'ai roulé ma bosse dans l'Europe de l'Est en faisant toute sorte de petits jobs.

I knocked about in Eastern Europe doing all kinds of odd jobs.

zoner

bum around, to go here and there, lit. walk in the zone

**Au lieu de zoner dans le quartier, tu ferais mieux d'aller
t'inscrire à l'A.N.P.E.**

*Instead of bumming around in the neighborhood, you would be
better off registering at the unemployment office.*

glander

to do nothing, from gland, acorn or head of the dick

J'vais peut-être glander à la maison.

I may just stay home and do nothing.

Or

to do

Qu'est-ce que tu glandes maintenant que t'es retraitée ?

What are you doing now that you're retired?

glandeur, glandeuse

good-for-nothing

Georges est un glandeur de première.

Georges is a real good-for-nothing.

se gratter les couilles

to have nothing to do, lit. to scratch one's balls

Depuis ce matin j'me gratte les couilles au bureau.

Since this morning, I've had nothing to do at work.

farniente, m

to do nothing, lit. to do nothing in Italian

**Le farniente est une activité prenante qui demande peu
de compétences.**

To do nothing is an activity that takes little skill.

ne rien ficher / foutre
to do nothing
Mon frère fiche rien de toute la journée.
My brother does nothing all day long.

ne pas en planter une
to do nothing, lit. to not plant any
Si t'es pas toujours derrière lui, Jason n'en plante pas une.
If you're not always behind him, Jason does nothing.

se la couler douce
to have it easy, lit. to flow it slowly
Quand je pense que mon ex-mari s'a coule douce aux Bermudes et que je dois travailler pour effacer nos dettes, ça me rend folle !
When I think that my ex-husband has it easy in Bermuda and I have to work to pay back our debts, it makes me crazy!

ne pas se fouler des masses / la rate
to not struggle, lit. to not strain masses (weight) / the spleen
T'inquiète, ils ont pas besoin de se fouler la rate pour réussir leurs études.
Don't worry, they don't have to struggle to do well in their studies.

fainéant, fainéante, feignasse, f,
slacker, lazybones, lit. who does nothing, fait néant
Va falloir que tu te débrouilles tout seul. Sors-toi les pouces du cul, feignasse!
You'll have to deal with that by yourself. Take your thumbs out of your ass, lazybones!

tire au flanc, m

slacker, lazybones

Il a tellement de talents mais aucune envie de les mettre à contribution. C'est un vrai tire au flanc.

He has so many talents but not a single desire to use them. He's a real slacker.

avoir les côtes en long

to be a lazybones, lit. to have the ribs placed vertically

Yves a rien fait de toute la semaine. Il a les côtes en long.

Yves did nothing all week long. He's a lazybones.

bonimenteur / baratineur, m

shark

Les bonimenteurs sont présents dans tous les marchés.

Sharks are present at all flea markets.

The family of *baratin* finds its origin in the word *barat*, trade or deal. *Baratiner* is to persuade someone to buy one's wares—even if of poor quality—thanks to one's above-average charm, exaggerations, and outright lies about the products. *Baratineurs* are also called *bonimenteurs*, a word that combines *boniment*, a sales talk or sweet talk, and *menteur*, liar. Though they once filled the streets and markets, *bonimenteurs* are nearly an extinct species; in-your-face advertising has taken their jobs away. The word is still present in the love field, a niche in which the same techniques are used to reach one's goal, this time for seduction rather than a salad spinner.

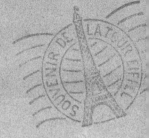

CHAPTER ELEVEN

Pleins les poches:
Shake Your Moneymaker

Prior to the euro, France used the *franc français* or *nouveau franc*. But switching to the euro was not the first time the French had been subjected to currency changes. In 1960, a painful change occurred when the *franc nouveau* replaced the *franc lourd*, which was then renamed the *franc ancien*. The exchange rate was easy; people had to divide the old price by 100 to arrive at the new one. Imagine how many millionaires in *francs lourds* suddenly became merely 'thousandaires'? But as with any big change, people were attached to their old ways and found the new currency difficult. Even TV journalists used both values to help people adapt to the conversion.

France witnessed the passage to the euro, the collective European Union currency, on January 1, 1999. The change came and the hype surrounding the euro created both fear and excitement in the general population. It's interesting to see that old people who have survived both monetary changes still speak in terms of the *franc ancien*!

Money has inspired plenty of slang words and popular expressions. Loved or despised, cash has left a lasting mark on the French language.

Cash

blé, m
dough, lit. wheat
On va se faire un max de blé sur ce deal.
We are going to make a lot of dough on this deal.

fric, m
cash, moolah
T'as le fric?
Have you got the cash?

pognon, m
money, from pogne, hand
Il est plein de pognon.
He's made of money.

flouze, m
money, Arabic word meaning money
Il veut du flouze mais veut pas bosser.
He wants money but doesn't want to work.

rond, m
dime, coin, lit. round
J't'aurais bien aidée mais j'ai plus un rond.
I'd help you out but I don't have a single dime.

radis, m
dime, lit. radish
Je n'ai plus un radis!
I don't have a dime.

balle, f
franc, lit. ball
Un étranger m'a demandé cent balles dans la rue.
A foreigner asked me for 100 francs in the street.

thune, f
five francs coin and money
T'as pas une thune?
Don't you have 5 francs?
Or
J'ai besoin de thunes.
I need money.

mitraille, f
coins, lit. scrap iron

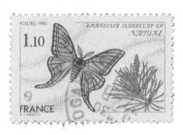

Les catholiques se débarrassent de leur mitraille à l'église.
Catholics get rid of their coins at church.

bifton, m
banknote, bill
File-moi un bifton.
Give me a banknote.

The Haves and Have-Nots

être râpe
to be stingy, cheap, lit. to be (like a) grater
T'es vraiment trop râpe—je dois toujours payer quand on sort ensemble.
You're really stingy—I always have to pay when we go out together.

finir sur la paille

to wind up in the poorhouse, lit. to finish on straw

Si on continue à dépenser autant d'argent, on va finir sur la paille.

If we continue to spend money like this, we're going to wind up in the poorhouse.

être fauché / à sec

to be flat broke, lit. to be moved / dry

Depuis mon deuxième divorce, je suis à sec.

Since my second divorce, I'm flat broke.

demander une rallonge

to ask for more (money, salary advance), lit. to ask for an extension

Si t'as pas assez d'argent pour finir le mois, demande une rallonge à ton patron.

If you don't have enough money to end the month, ask your boss for a salary advance.

joindre les deux bouts

to make ends meet

Avec son salaire de vendeuse, Aurélie peut pas joindre les deux bouts.

With her cashier's salary, Aurélie can't make ends meet.

faire la manche

to beg for money, lit. to do the sleeve

Le métro de Paris est plein de Gitanes qui font la manche.

The Paris métro is filled with Gypsies who beg for money.

être dans le rouge
to be in the red
Dix minutes à Vegas et j'étais 200 balles dans le rouge.
Ten minutes in Vegas and I was 200 bucks in the red.

être plein aux as
to be made of money, lit. to be full of aces
Mon ami d'uni est plein aux as.
My friend from college is made of money.

être friqué
to be loaded, from fric, money
Noah n'a pas un sou; c'est sa femme qui est friquée.
Noah has no money; his wife is loaded.

avoir les reins solides
to have enough money, lit. to have solid kidneys
Ne t'inquiète pas, j'ai les reins solides.
Don't worry; I have enough money.

se faire des couilles en or
to make a fortune, lit. to make one's balls golden
**Si notre entreprise fonctionne, on va s'faire des
    couilles en or.**
If our business works, we're going make a fortune.

se remplir les fouilles
to fill one's pockets, lit. to fill up the excavations
**Pendant que les travailleurs se cassent le cul, les
    actionnaires se remplissent les fouilles.**
*While the workers break their asses, the stockholders fill their
    pockets.*

avoir les poches trouées

to be a big spender, lit. to have pockets with holes

Ne lui confie pas tout l'argent, ta femme a les poches trouées.

Don't let your wife be responsible for all the money; she's a big spender.

claquer

to waste, lit. to flap

Il a claqué son fric au cabaret.

He wasted his dough at the cabaret.

flamber

to burn, lit. to blaze

Les enfants riches flambent le flouze de leurs parents.

Rich kids burn their parents' money.

flambeur, flambeuse

big spender, lit. burner

Quel flambeur! Bernard a claqué 20'000 euro.

What a big spender! Bernard wasted 20,000 euros.

toucher le jackpot / le Pactole

to hit the jackpot

Alice rêve de toucher le Pactole au casino.

Alice dreams of hitting the jackpot at the casino.

Pactole is the name of a river containing a lot of gold in the ancient kingdom of Crésus. The French also say someone is *riche comme Crésus*, meaning very wealthy.

Cost of Living

taxer
to be expensive, lit. to tax
Ça taxe, cette paire de pompes!
This pair of shoes is expensive!

France is known for having painfully high taxes. Luckily, it is only a stone's throw from several fiscal paradises: Luxembourg, Switzerland, and Monaco. Think the IRS is bad? The French equivalent, the *Fisc,* is known to create fear even in the eyes of the country's most powerful. Many artists, athletes, and CEOs and the headquarters of big industries have moved to Switzerland or Luxembourg to save a few bucks. In France, as in the rest of the world, people have different monetary philosophies. Some work to live while others live to work. Not all the rich have left France—they abound on the Champs-Elysées for example. But in addition to being envied, the rich are also the target of insults. Note these commonly used expressions:

Il vaut mieux être pauvre et en bonne santé que riche et malade.
(Better to be poor and in good health than rich and sick.)
This is a play on the classic proverb:
Il vaut mieux être riche et en bonne santé que pauvre et malade.
(Better to be rich and in good health than poor and sick.)

douiller

to be expensive, lit. to shell out
Le resto est bon, mais putain ça douille!
The restaurant is good, but it's f**king expensive.

casser les prix

to have discount prices, lit. to break prices
Les supermarchés cassent les prix.
Supermarkets have discount prices.

prendre l'ascenseur

to rise quickly, lit. to take the elevator
Le prix de l'essence prend l'ascenseur.
The price of gasoline is rising quickly.

prix plancher, m

lowest price, lit. price that touches the floor
Tous les articles sont vendus au prix plancher.
All the articles are sold at the lowest prices.

être donné

to be cheap, lit. to be given
À vingt euro par nuit, cet hôtel est donné.
At twenty euros a night, this hotel is cheap.

coûter la peau du cul

to cost an arm and a leg, lit. to cost the skin of the ass
Une robe de mariage de couturier peut coûter la peau du cul.
A designer wedding dress can cost an arm and a leg.

CHAPTER TWELVE

Garde ou voleur?:
The Wrong Side of the Law

Chances are you won't stray to the wrong side of the law in France. But if you do, don't expect an Inspector Clouseau or detective Hercule Poirot (Belgian, actually) to prove your innocence. French *flics* have a reputation about as good as the LAPD's. Last thing you want to do is wake your Grandma up at midnight to tell her you're in a French prison and need to be bailed out. Unless, of course, you're eager to spend 24 hours sitting in a cell. It's preferable to remain sitting down, if you know what we mean—getting up is as risky in French jails as in American jails.

Drugs don't seem to be as big a problem in France as in the US, but you'll still see your fair share of addicts roaming the streets after dark. Marijuana smoking is extremely common and it's likely to be the only drug you witness firsthand in France. That is, if you don't consider the national drugs of cigarettes and alcohol. Old French drunks are quite a sight, stumbling around with their pants undone, attempting to pee on a *mur* or beautiful old building. What is considered public indecency in the US is the norm here: Men unzip and urinate anywhere and everywhere. If only it were that easy for the *demoiselles* . . .

Tabac et Autre Drogues

To fight *le tabagisme passif*, secondhand smoke, February 1, 2007, marked the prohibition of smoking in all schools, restaurants, bars, indoor public places, and waiting areas. This measure was to be followed on January 1, 2008, by the interdiction of smoke in *bar-tabacs*, *discothèques*, and nightclubs. The dangerous level of smoke in these places is usually higher than on the smoggiest day in Paris, when children and old people are kindly asked to stay home or wear a mask!

accro, m, f

addicted, junky, lit. the hanged one, from accrocher to hang
Les accros au tabac en France vont devoir fumer dehors.
Tobacco addicts in France will have to smoke outside.

sèche, f

smoke, lit. a dry one
Hugo est sorti s'acheter un paquet de sèches.
Hugo went out to buy a package of smokes.

clope, f

ciggy, smoke
File moi une clope, je suis à sec.
Give me a smoke; I'm all out.

bedos, m

joint, from the Romani
T'as assez fumé. Fais tourner le bedos !
You've smoked enough. Pass the joint!

pétard / joint, m
spliff, lit. a firecracker / joint
Après un pétard, ma cousine dansait sur les tables.
After a spliff, my cousin was dancing on the tables.

herbe, f, beuh in verlan
weed, pot, lit. grass
Après une taffe d'herbe, Benoît était stone.
After a hit of weed, Benoît was stoned.

Drugs contain a wealth of slang expressions. Clearly property of the street, drugs had to be given other names and their own vocabulary to avoid drawing unwanted attention. Once understandable only by those in the know, this talk has now become extremely common. Although all illicit drugs are illegal in France, the police will often tolerate a small amount of marijuana per person, assuming that it is for personal use only. However, be warned that any and all drug possession can mean jail time, even for American tourists who declare, "*Je ne savais pas!*"

chichon, m
hash, abbr. from hashish, Arabic word
Si tu vois Luke, demande-lui un peu de chichon.
If you see Luke, ask him for a bit of hash.

fumer une canne
to smoke a joint, lit. to smoke a canne
Des élèves ont fumé une cane dans les toilettes.
Some students smoked a joint in the toilets.

cône, m
spliff, lit. a cone
Rouler un cône demande un certain savoir-faire.
Rolling a spliff takes a certain amount of know-how.

planer
to be high, lit. to sailplane
**En mélangeant médicaments, alcool et joints, Coralie et
Steve planaient trop grave hier soir.**
*Mixing medication, alcohol, and weed, Coralie and Steve
were too high last night.*

came, camelote, f
drugs, lit. junk
**Les gros trafiquants livrent leur camelote aux
revendeurs.**
Big drug traffickers deliver their junk to dealers.

sniff, f
snuff, from sniffer, to inhale
Ils se sont mis dans le nez 200 dollars de sniff.
They put 200 dollars of snuff up their noses.

tox, toxico, m, f
drug addict, abbr. of toxicomane
Les toxicos traînent dans le parc.
Drug addicts hang out in the park.

être stone / défoncé
to be stoned / demolished
Mark a besoin de plus que ça pour être stone.
Mark needs more than that to be stoned.

The Players

flic, m / flicaille, f

cop, pig, from the German, Fliege, fly

Les flics m'ont arrêté dans la rue sans raison.

The cops stopped me in the street for no reason.

poulet, m

cop, lit. chicken

Un poulet nous suit depuis plus de dix minutes.

A cop has been following us for ten minutes.

condé, m

cop, verlan for des cons

Les condés en civil assurent la sécurité des vols.

Plainclothes cops provide flight security.

ripou, verlan for pourri

corrupt cop, lit. rotten

Les dealers ont été informés par un ripou.

Dealers were informed by a corrupt cop.

The term *ripou,* verlan for *pourri,* was popularized by the movie *Les Ripoux,* directed by Claude Zidi. Staring Phillipe Noiret and a young Thierry Lhermitte, it became a cult movie of the 1980s. The sequel, *Ripoux contre ripoux* or *Ripoux 2,* was released in 1990, and 2003 saw a series comeback with *Les Ripoux 3.* Filled with bad language, worse manners, corruption, and talented actors, the series has found a treasured place in French cinematic history.

taupe, f

spy, lit. mole (the animal)

Les services secrets français ont des taupes partout.

The French secret service has spies everywhere.

caïd, m

gang chief, from the Arabic

La police recherche le caïd de la cité.

Police are looking for the gang chief of the city.

petite frappe, f

gangbanger, lit. little slap

Les petites frappes de la cité effraient les mémés.

The city's gangbangers frighten old ladies.

revendeur, m

dealer, lit. re-seller

Un revendeur m'a abordé dans la rue.

A dealer accosted me in the street.

chiper / tirer

to steal, from Latin *capere*, to take / pull

Yasser a chipé le sac à main de Marlène.

Yasser stole Marlène's purse.

choper

to take, to catch, from Latin *capere*, to take / pull

L'enseignant a chopé les élèves qui trichaient.

The teacher caught the students who were cheating.

tauper
to steal, from taupe, mole
Frédéric a perdu son job au fast-food car il taupait dans la caisse.
Frédéric lost his job at the fast-food joint because he stole from the cash register.

en cavale
on the run, from cheval, horse
Les terroristes sont toujours en cavale.
The terrorists are still on the run.

pris en flag / pris la main dans le sac
to be caught red-handed, abbr. of flagrant délit / lit. hand caught in the purse
Le voleur a été pris la main dans le sac.
The thief was caught red-handed.

pincer / serrer
to arrest, lit. to pinch / to grip
La police a pincé l'escroc.
The police caught the hood.

être en GAV
to be in custody, abbr. of garde à vue, custody
Le suspect est en GAV.
The suspect is in custody.

pot-de-vin, m
bribe, lit. pitcher of wine
Le maire a reçu des pots-de-vin.
The mayor took bribes.

dessous de table, m

bribe, lit. (money received from) under the table

Il a dû toucher un dessous de table pour délivrer ce permis de construire!

He must have taken a bribe to deliver this building permit.

magouiller

to fix, from magouille, scheme

Les résultats des élections ont été magouillées.

The results of the elections were fixed.

magouilleur, magouilleuse

schemer

Le comptable de ma boîte est un magouilleur de premier ordre.

The accountant of my company is a very good schemer.

combine, f

trick, abbr. of combinaison, recipe

J'ai trouvé une combine pour gagner un max de fric en peu de temps.

I found a trick to win a lot of money in a short time.

se faire embobiner

to be duped, lit. to be put on a bobbin

Christine s'est faite embobinée par l'habile vendeur de voitures d'occasion. Elle a payé $10,000 pour un vrai tacot.

Christine was duped by the slick used-car salesman. She paid $10,000 for a real lemon.

pigeon, m

someone who got ripped off, lit. a pigeon

T'as acheté ce cendrier pour quinze euro? T'es un pigeon!

You bought this ashtray for fifteen euros? You got ripped off!

Pigeons aren't only in Piazza San Marco, Venice, Italy. The French monuments attract many of these feathered visitors, as well as tourists who swarm the souvenir shops. Always crowding monuments, parks, and public places, especially in August, tourists act much like birds attracted by breadcrumbs. What better term than *pigeon* to describe them! As an extension of this principle, the term *pigeon* is now used for any customer who gets duped in a deal.

plumer qqn

to rip someone off, lit. to pluck someone

Serges a son propre magasin et il adore plumer les gens.

Serges has his own store and loves to rip people off.

Weapons and Criminals

pétard, m

gun, lit. firecracker

Je faisais la queue à la banque lorsque la personne devant moi a sorti un pétard et a crié: « C'est un hold up! Personne ne bouge! »

I was standing in line at the bank when the person in front of me took out a gun and yelled: "This is a holdup! Nobody move!"

flingue, m
piece, lit. stick

Depuis qu'il a été tabassé, Nicolas ne sort plus sans son flingue.

Since he was beat up, Nicolas doesn't go out without his piece anymore.

flinguer
to gun down, lit. from flingue, gun

« Si tu bouges je te flingue » a crié le policier en brandissant son arme de service.

"If you move I'll gun you down," cried the policeman while brandishing his service weapon.

se flinguer
to shoot oneself, from flingue, gun

Il devait être vachement déprimé pour se flinguer.

He must have been really depressed to shoot himself.

Although crime rates are rising, the French feel no need to have guns at home in order to ensure their own safety. You won't find bullets at corner stores and if you do find them, you will need far more than a valid driver's license to purchase and possess a weapon. While your biggest risk as a tourist is an armed mugging, for the more than 5,000 American children who die each year from firearms, similar restrictions could mean the difference between life and death. Don't take your gun with you, cowboy! France is not a dangerous place to live or visit; the worst that'll happen is you'll get mugged in the *métro*.

saigner qqn

to bleed someone

Si tu t'approches encore je vais te saigner comme un porc.

If you come any closer I'm going to bleed you like a pig.

surin, m

knife, from the Romani

Le mec a sorti un surin et a menacé Damien de le tuer s'il ne lui donnait pas son argent.

A guy took out a knife, threatened to kill Damien if he didn't give him his money.

surineur, m

killer (who uses a knife)

Le surineur attend sa victime, dans l'ombre, au fond de la rue.

The killer waits for his victim, in the shadow, at the end the street.

butter

to kill, lit. to hit an obstacle

« Si vous criez ou bougez, je vous butte » a dit le terroriste à ses otages.

"If you scream or move, I'll kill you," said the terrorist to his hostages.

bousiller

to destroy, lit. to do a shitty job, from bouse, cow shit

Notre chat a bousillé tous nos meubles.

Our cat destroyed all our furniture.

refroidir qqn

to kill someone, lit. to chill someone

Le kidnappeur a menacé de refroidir l'enfant si les parents avertissent la police.

The kidnapper threatened to kill the child if the parents called the police.

placard, m, carpla in verlan

jail, lit. cabinet

Mike a fait cinq ans de carpla.

Mike spent five years in jail.

taule, f

jail, lit. home

Pedro finira en taule, c'est moi qui vous le dis.

Pedro will end up in jail, I'm telling you.

mitard, m

jail, from *mite*

Au mitard, le petit voleur a appris comment améliorer sa technique.

In jail, the smalltime thief learned how to improve his technique.

au frais / à l'ombre

in the slammer, lit. in the fresh air / shade

Le violeur va passer quelques années à l'ombre.

The rapist is going to spend a few years in the slammer.

se faire la belle / se faire la malle

to escape, lit. to make one's nice one / to make one's trunk

Deux taulards se sont fait la belle.

Two prisoners escaped.

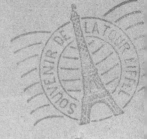

CHAPTER THIRTEEN

Toubib or not toubib:
Following Doctor's Orders

No one expects to *tomber malade*, on their travels in France. Besides a slight case of the runs from all that wonderfully creamy *fromage* you'll eat, there's no real medical risk to visiting the country. But if you do fall ill, know that you are in safe hands. France's top-notch healthcare system is one of the world's best. *La Sécurité Sociale*, affectionately known as *la Sécu*, is the government system that acts as an insurance, assuring the healthcare costs of every single person living in France. When someone can't meet the requirements for *la Sécu*, they are covered 100 percent free under *CMU, couverture maladie universelle*. Whether you're young or old, rich or poor, underemployed or out of a job, you've got health insurance.

Unlike Britain's National Health Service, France does not have a system of traditional socialized medicine. Rather, the French system works with private insurers and doctors who all accept *la Sécu*'s health insurance plan. The French are allowed to choose their own doctors and specialists, without any need for approval beforehand. The beauty of this system is that there are no long waiting lists like in the UK, and average folks totally control their own healthcare, picking and choosing doctors as they wish. The government trusts its citizens not to abuse the system and so far it has worked. Envious yet?

Health

avoir une pêche d'enfer
to feel like a million bucks, lit. to have a peach from Hell
J'ai vu Géraldine à midi. Elle a une pêche d'enfer!
I saw Géraldine at noon. She feels like a million bucks today!

carburer à qqch
to run on something, lit. to fuel up
Tu carbures au café pour être autant excité?
Do you run on coffee to be so excited?

tenir le coup
to make it, lit. to hold on
Le mec de Tina l'a larguée y a une semaine. Elle tient bien le coup.
Tina's boyfriend dumped her a week ago. She's holding on.

ne pas avoir la frite
to not feel so hot, lit. to not have the French fry
Carole, t'as pas l'air d'avoir la frite.
Carole, you don't look like you feel so hot.

ne pas être dans son assiette
to not seem like oneself, lit. not to be in one's dish
Qu'est-ce qui t'est arrivé? T'as pas l'air dans ton assiette.
What happened to you? You don't seem like yourself.

coup de pompe / barre

to get very tired, lit. hit of pump

Myriam a eu un coup de pompe et est rentrée chez elle.

Myriam got very tired and went back home.

être crevé

be dead (tired), lit. to be burst

Après une journée de travail, les ouvriers sont crevés.

After a day's work, the laborers are dead.

être à bout de souffle

to be out of breath/exhausted, lit. to be at the end of breath

Après avoir couru dix km, elle était à bout de souffle.

After having run ten km, she was exhausted.

Life and Death

No need to say that every person who enjoys life is afraid of death. As Woody Allen, beloved by the French, attests, "I am not afraid of death; I just don't want to be there when it happens." All the vocabulary around this frightening topic is either ironic or purposefully distant, alluding to death using random and often bizarre images.

caner

to die, lit. to abandon

Sa grand-mère va bientôt caner.

His grandmother is going to die soon.

claquer

to die, lit. to flap

La fille de Sarah lui a claqué dans les bras.

Sarah's daughter died in her arms.

sortir les pieds devant

to leave a place in a coffin, lit. to go out feet first

Mon grand-père est sorti de l'hôpital les pieds devant.

My grandfather left the hospital in a coffin.

casser sa pipe

to kick the bucket, lit. to break one's pipe

Des soldats cassent leur pipe pour rien.

Soldiers kick the bucket for nothing.

manger les pissenlits par la racine

bite the dust, lit. to eat dandelions from the root

Les anti-végétariens finissent eux aussi par manger les pissenlits par la racine.

Anti-vegetarians also bite the dust.

lit. Anti-vegetarians also finish up eating dandelions by the root.

boulevard des allongés, m

cemetery, lit. the boulevard of the (people) lying down

Mon cousin a pris un studio au boulevard des allongés.

My cousin died.

lit. My cousin took a studio on the boulevard of the lying down.

frôler la mort

to have a brush with death, lit. to brush against death

Le cascadeur a frôlé la mort.

The stuntman had a brush with death.

sentir le sapin

to smell like death, lit. to smell pine

Ça sent le sapin dans cette maison de vieux.

It smells like death in this old folks' home.

être au bout du rouleau

to be at the end of one's days, to be exhausted, lit. to be at the
end of the roll

Mon ami est au bout du rouleau.

My friend is at the end of his days.

Birth

prendre la pilule

to take the pill

**Désolée, j'aurais dû t' dire plus tôt que j'prends pas la
pilule.**

Sorry, I should've told you beforehand that I don't take the pill.

se faire enfler

to get pregnant, lit. to get inflated

Diane s'est faite enfler lors de ses vacances en Turquie.

Diane got pregnant during her vacation in Turkey.

avoir le ballon / le gros bide

to show (during pregnancy), lit. to have a balloon / a big belly

**Irina n'a pas encore le ballon, mais elle est enceinte de
cinq mois.**

Irina isn't showing yet, but she's five months pregnant.

mettre qqn en cloque

to knock somebody up, lit. to put somebody in lump

**Ça fait pas deux mois que Jean a fait la connaissance
de Sofia et il l'a déjà mise en cloque.**

*It hasn't been two months since Jean met Sofia and he has
already knocked her up.*

avoir un polichinelle dans le tiroir

to be pregnant, lit. to have a marionette in the drawer

**Je reconnais à peine Adeline depuis qu'elle a un pol-
ichinelle dans le tiroir.**

I hardly recognize Adeline since she got pregnant

être enceinte jusqu'à l'os

to be pregnant, lit. to be pregnant to the bone

**Non, Josette n'est pas en retard sur son cycle, elle est
enceinte jusqu'à l'os.**

No, Josette isn't just late, she's pregnant.

With the second highest birthrate in Europe, France
certainly needs many slang expressions for pregnancy.
French women have an average of 1.89 children, which
doesn't meet the 2.1 required to maintain a stable population rate, but comes awfully close.

The reason for this seems to lie in France's unique
blend of work and family. In France, families receive an
allowance for every child, plus a large bonus for the third
child. *Les crèches*, day care centers, are sponsored by the
government. The perks do not stop there—French women
are offered generous monetary incentives, around $1,000 a
month, to stay home instead of working for one year after
their third child is born.

While all this seems plausible, Dirty French has
another theory: French women are simply unable to resist
Frenchmen, known as the world's best lovers.

Pain

bobo, m
cut, boo-boo
Tu vas pas aller aux urgences pour ce petit bobo!
You won't go to the ER for this little boo-boo!

s'en sortir
to heal, to get better, lit. to come out of it
Ne te fais pas de soucis, ton ami va s'en sortir.
Don't worry, your friend will get better.

crever de mal
to die of pain
**En fermant la porte de la voiture, Benjamin s'est arra-
ché un ongle et crève de mal.**
*Closing the car door, Benjamin lost a fingernail and is now
dying of pain.*

avoir mal au caillou
to have a headache, lit. to have pain in the stone
T'as pas de l'aspirine? J'ai trop mal au caillou.
You don't have an aspirin, do you? I've got such a headache.

être bouillant (de fièvre)
to be boiling (with fever)
Amène ton fils aux urgences, il est bouillant.
Bring your son to the ER; he's boiling.

légume, m
vegetable
Mon père préfère mourir que finir en légume.
My father prefers to die than to end up a vegetable.

choper froid / la crève

to catch a cold

Nous avons chopé la crève en montagne.

We caught a cold in the mountains.

choper une saloperie

to catch a nasty disease lit. to get a dirty thing

Christophe a chopé une saloperie en Thaïlande.

Christophe caught a nasty disease in Thailand.

MST, f

STD, abbr. of Maladie Sexuellement Transmissible

**L'abstinence est la meilleure protection contre les MST
et le plaisir sexuel.**

*Abstinence is the best way to avoid an STD as well as sexual
pleasure.*

SIDA, sida, m

AIDS, abbr. of Syndrome d'Immuno Déficience Acquise

Tu vas pas choper le sida en me parlant.

You won't get AIDS by talking to me.

Doctors

prendre un médoc

to take some medicine

Au lieu de souffrir de tes allergies, prends un médoc!

Instead of suffering from your allergies, take some medicine!

hosto, m

hospital, abbr. of hôpital

On a dû amener Sacha à l'hosto.

We had to bring Sacha to the hospital.

toubib, m, f

doc, from the Arabic

Le toubib de Greg lui a conseillé de toujours employer des capotes pour éviter les maladies sexuelles.

Greg's doc advised him to always use rubbers to avoid sexually transmitted diseases.

physio, m, f

physical therapist, abbr. of physiothérapeute

Je dois aller voir un physio au plus vite.

I need to go see a physical therapist as soon as possible.

guigne trou, m, f

gyno, lit. hole-peeker, from guigner, to peek

Chaque année, les femmes devraient aller voir leur guigne trou.

Each year, women should go see their gynos.

zieutiste, m, f

eye doctor, from zieuter, to look

Le zieutiste dit que Mike doit porter des lunettes.

The eye doctor says that Mike needs to wear glasses.

tranche-lard, m

surgeon, lit. the one who cuts the bacon

J'veux pas finir entre les mains de ce vieux tranche-lard.

I don't want to end up in that old surgeon's hands.

passer sur le billard

to have an operation, lit. to pass on the billiards

Diana a les jetons. Elle passe sur le billard.

Diana is scared. She's having an operation.

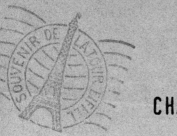

CHAPTER FOURTEEN

Guerre et paix:
Looking for Trouble and Keeping the Peace

If there is a major difference between the US and France, it can be found in their opposing attitudes toward war. Once a *guerrier* country—remember a tiny man named Napoléon?—France has lately chosen the camp of *la paix* and diplomacy. For the refusal to enter the coalition against Iraq and other recent adventures into war, French products were boycotted in the US, where some Americans chose to ditch the *Camembert* and *Bordeaux* until France gave in. If the war in Iraq had only lasted a year or so, perhaps the French could've understood giving these things up for that short time. Half a decade later, though, most French don't agree—Dirty French dares you to take away a French person's favorite cheese and wine for that long—expect WW III, and that's if you're lucky!

Napoléon, perhaps the most famed *Français* of all time after *Inspecteur Clouseau*, tried to conquer Europe and expand *l'empire français*. More than a simple conquering of territory, Napoléon attempted to bring French culture to the rest of heathen Europe.

Dirty French doesn't understand why they weren't thankful for this effort. If you've ever eaten at a *restaurant* in Poland or sipped a bottle of Swiss wine, you'll certainly agree with us.

In present-day France, fights are caused by only a handful of topics: food, drink, sports, political speech, and the police. With this in mind, the same attitude of avoiding interpersonal conflict can be found in many Dirty French expressions. Spoken in a good tone with the correct body language, simple words can save you a lot of pain, medical care, and expensive plastic surgery.

Annoyances

chercher midi à quatorze heures

to make something more complicated, lit. to look for noon at 2 pm

Ne cherche pas midi à quatorze heures. Y a rien besoin de modifier, la lettre est déjà parfaite!

Don't look for a needle in a haystack. There's no need to modify anything; the letter is already perfect!

chercher qqn

to be looking for trouble, lit. to seek someone

Ce petit con me cherche depuis le début de la soirée.

This little jerk has been looking for trouble with me since the beginning of the evening.

chercher des poux / la petite bête

to ask for trouble, lit. to look for lice / for the small beast

Tu m'cherches des poux maintenant?

Are you asking me for trouble now?

chercher la baston / la rixe

to look for a fight, lit. to look for a stick / fight

J'cherche pas la baston, mon gars; j'te dis qu'j'aimerais bien baiser ta meuf.

I'm not looking for a fight, dude, I'm just saying that I'd like to f**k your girlfriend.

chercher la castagne, f

to look for a fight, lit. to look for a chestnut (slang for punch)

Mon voisin a cherché la castagne et m'a trouvé sur son chemin.

My neighbor looked for trouble and found me in his path.

pomper l'air

to really annoy, lit. to pump the air away

Maman, tu me pompes l'air avec tes mises en garde; j'ai presque 30 ans.

You really annoy me with your warnings, mom; I'm almost 30.

casser les couilles

to break someone's balls

Arrête de me casser les couilles avec cette histoire. Je t'ai dit que j'en ai rien à foutre!

Stop breaking my balls with that story. I told you I don't give a shit about it!

trouer le cul à qqn

to get on someone's nerves, lit. to make a hole in someone's ass

Ta gueule! Là, tu commences grave à me trouer le cul.

Shut up! Now, you're starting to really get on my nerves.

ne pas lâcher les baskets à qqn

to be on someone's case, lit. to not let go of someone's
sneakers

**Pour recevoir une pension alimentaire plus importante,
l'ex de Bernard lui a plus lâché les baskets.**

*To get more child support, Bernard's ex-wife was continuously
on his case.*

avoir sa claque de qqn / qqch

to have had it up to here with someone / something, lit. to
have one's slap with someone / something

Yvan a eu sa claque de toi et de ta mauvaise humeur.

Yvan has had it up to here with you and your bad mood.

coller qqn

to stick to somebody like glue, to follow somebody closely

**Arianne, ton copain a besoin d'air! Arrête de le coller
en permanence!**

*Arianne, your boyfriend needs air! Stop sticking to him like
glue!*

lâcher la grappe à qqn

to leave someone alone, lit. to let go of one's bunch

**Si mes collègues pouvaient me lâcher la grappe pen-
dant une heure, ce serait le paradis.**

*If my colleagues could leave me alone for one hour, it would
be heaven.*

faire chier / caguer qqn

to annoy someone, lit. to make someone shit

Tu m'dis si j'te fais chier.

Tell me if I'm annoying you.

se faire chier

to be bored, lit. to make oneself shit

Comme j'me suis fait chier en vacances; j'étais en Bretagne et il a plu tous les jours.

How bored I was during my vacation; I was in Brittany and it rained every day.

blairer qqn / sentir qqn

to stand someone, lit. to smell someone

Après que sa copine l'a trompé, Marek pouvait plus la blairer et est parti.

After his girlfriend cheated on him, Marek couldn't stand her anymore and left.

Peacekeeping

la fermer / fermer sa gueule

to shut up, lit. to close it, to close one's mouth

Elisa ferait mieux de fermer sa grosse gueule ou Patrice va s'énerver grave.

Elisa had better shut up or Patrice is going to get really angry.

se casser / se tirer

to leave, lit. to break / pull oneself

Si tu veux mon conseil, casse-toi!

If you want my advice, just leave!

se barrer

to get out, to take off, lit. to dam oneself

Barrons-nous de ce bar; il va y avoir une descente de police!

Let's get out of this bar; the police will be here soon!

foutre le camp

to take off, lit. to leave the camp

Lorsque les pickpockets ont vu la voiture de police, ils ont vite foutu le camp.

When the pickpockets saw the police car, they quickly took off.

aller voir ailleurs (si j'y suis)

to leave someone alone, lit. to go see somewhere else (if I'm there)

Écoute gamin, je suis en train de parler avec ta mère, alors va voir ailleurs si j'y suis!

Listen kid, I'm speaking with your mom; so leave me alone!

s'occuper de ses oignons

to mind one's own business, lit. to take care of one's onions

Occupe-toi de tes oignons; laisse-le se débrouiller.

Mind your own business; let him deal with it.

ramener sa fraise

to butt in, lit. to bring one's strawberry (fraise is slang for head)

Arrête de ramener ta fraise, c'est chiant.

Stop butting in, that's annoying.

se mettre qqch où je pense

to shove it, lit. to put it where I'm thinking (in the ass)

Ton avis tu peux te le mettre où je pense.

Take your advice and shove it.

aller se faire voir / cuire un œuf

to take a hike, lit. to go show oneself cook oneself an egg

Si tu le prends comme ça, va te faire cuire un œuf!

If you take it like that, take a hike!

aller se faire foutre (chez les Grecs)
to go f**k oneself, lit. to go get f**ked (by Greeks)
Pays de merde, allez tous vous faire foutre!
F**king country, go f**k yourselves!

aller chier dans sa caisse
to take a hike, lit. to go shit in one's box
**T'es gentille mais tu nous déranges là; alors va chier
dans ta caisse!**
*You're nice but you're disturbing us right now; so go
take a hike!*

ficher / foutre la paix à qqn
to leave someone in peace
**Fous-moi la paix une bonne fois
pour toutes.**
Leave me in peace once and for all.

Fighting

engueuler
to shout at someone, from gueule, mouth
**Le patron a engueulé ses employés lors du souper de
compagnie.**
The boss shouted at his employees during the company dinner.

casser la gueule à qqn
to kick, lit. to break someone's face
**Une bande de jeunes a cassé la gueule de Matthieu
dans le métro.**
A gang of youths kicked Matthieu in the subway.

se péter sur la gueule

to fight, lit. to explode on the face

Au lieu de vous péter sur la gueule, vous devriez prendre du temps et vous expliquer.

Instead of fighting, you should take some time to explain yourselves.

rouer de coups qqn

to beat someone black and blue, lit. to roll someone in punches

Des jeunes bourges ont roué de coups un vieux clodo.

Some young rich kids beat an old bum black and blue.

passer à tabac qqn / tabasser

to beat the shit out of someone

La police a passé à tabac le suspect qui ne voulait pas avouer.

The police beat the shit out of the suspect who wouldn't confess.

refaire le portrait de qqn

to destroy someone's face, lit. to redo someone's portrait

En se promenant de nuit à Berlin, mon cousin s'est fait refaire le portrait par une bande de skinheads.

While walking around in Berlin late at night, my cousin had his face bashed in by group of skinheads.

baston, f

fight, from bastonner, to hit with a stick

Y a eu une baston au bistro à cause du match de foot.

There was a fight at the bar due to the football game.

claque, f
slap, from an onomatopoeia
Ma mère m'a foutu une claque.
My mother slapped me.

tarte / patate, f
blow, lit. a pie / patate
Alice s'est prise une tarte en pleine poire.
Alice got a blow in the face.

tomber dans les pommes
to fall unconscious, lit. to fall in the apples
**Après avoir reçu un coup dans la gueule, Johann est
  tombé dans les pommes.**
After he got punched in the face, Johann fell unconscious.

envoyer qqn au tapis
to knock out someone, lit. to send someone to the carpet
**Le match de boxe venait de commencer quand le chal-
  lenger a été envoyé au tapis par le tenant du titre.**
*The boxing match had just started when the challenger was
  knocked out by the title holder.*

coup de boule, m
head-butt, lit. a hit of the ball (head)
D'un coup de boule, le footballeur a vengé son honneur.
With a head-butt, the footballer avenged his honor.

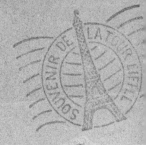

CHAPTER FIFTEEN

C'est trop ouf:
Life Is a Cabaret . . . or
Discothèque . . . or Brothel

Going out in France can come in many forms. You may spend a Saturday night at a giant *discothèque*, pumping electronic and techno until the wee hours of the morning. You may also choose to relax at an outdoor *café*, sipping *Bordeaux* while staring into the eyes of someone you love. If that doesn't work for you, maybe you'll head to a *cabaret* or nightclub, and chat with the strippers and hookers that call these seedy places home.

It's a sad truth that many prostitutes are exploited by their customers and pimps, but it seems impossible to eradicate *le plus vieux métier du monde*. In France, prostitution is neither illegal nor immoral. Strongly discouraged, it is looked at as a woman's right, even a last resort to going hungry. Authorities don't punish the customers or the prostitutes, as long as they are above the legal age for consent, aren't illegal immigrants, and pay taxes on their income. What's more, sex in France is considered the domain of one's private life, and is nobody's business. If a man pays for sex and if a woman earns a few bucks doing it, the French may make a disparaging remark but otherwise ignore the situation. You can imagine French disbelief during the Monica Lewinsky scandal. . . . Why on earth would anyone care who the president goes to bed with? they wondered. And further, why wasn't his sexual creativity (cigar, anyone?) applauded?

boxon, boucan m
noise, lit. brothel
Arrêtez ce boxon!
Stop that noise!

> *Boucan and boxon* were used for cabarets and brothels. These words derive from *bouc*, the male goat known as the Christian representation of Satan. Nowadays, those terms are only used as slang words for noise.

bordel, m
mess, brothel
C'est quoi ce bordel?
What's this mess?
or
Ils sortent du bordel.
They are coming out of the brothel.

pute, putain, f
whore, hooker, from the Latin putere, to stink
La plupart des putes en France sont africaines.
Most whores in France are African.

belle de nuit, f

lady of the night, lit. beauty of the night

Les belles de nuit se voient rarement de jour.

Ladies of the nights are rarely seen by day.

faire le tapin / tapiner

to prostitute oneself

Je ne vais quand même pas faire le tapin pour payer un loyer pareil!

I'm not going to prostitute myself to pay such a high rent!

The *tapin* family finds its roots in a small *tambour* that makes a lot of noise and was usually played in the streets.

Prostitution is no longer permitted on the street and in public places. A former law trying to eradicate sexual slavery closed all the brothels but recently the authorities discussed reopening them. *La maison close, le bordel,* and *le lupanar* (from Italian *lupa*, she-wolf) may come back, under the euphemistic appellation *le club*.

---

pince-cul, pince-fesse, m

cabaret/nightclub, lit. ass pincher

T'as encore passé la nuit dans un pince-fesse toi!

Once again you spent the night in a cabaret!

Entertainment

s'éclater

to have a lot of fun, lit. to blow oneself up

On va tous s'éclater au bord de la mer.

We'll all have a lot of fun at the seaside.

teuf, m

party, verlan for fête, party

Des voisins se sont plaints du bruit de la teuf.

Neighbors complained about the noise of the party.

faire la bamboula / la fiesta / la java

to party, words of foreign influence, Africa, Spain, Indonesia

On a fait la bamboula toute la nuit.

We partied all night long.

videur, m

bouncer, from vider, to empty

Ce videur use trop ses muscles et pas assez son cerveau.

This bouncer uses his muscles too much and his brain not enough.

gorille, m

bodyguard, lit. a gorilla

Le patron est toujours accompagné d'un gorille.

The boss is always accompanied by a bodyguard.

délit de sale gueule, m

discrimination based on one's face or skin color, lit. the crime of dirty face

Le délit de sale gueule est fréquent à l'entrée des discothèques.

Discrimination based on one's looks is frequent at discothèque entrances.

The *délit de sale gueule* occurs not only at discothèque entrances but also in the streets. On a slow day, policemen may judge ordinary citizens by their appearance or skin color, and ask to see their passport, identity card or worse, *le papier de séjour,* the French equivalent for the green card. But don't worry, if you don't look Arab or African, if you don't have a beard, if you don't wear hip-hop clothes, and if you don't speak French with a foreign accent then you shouldn't have a problem. Otherwise you may consider a visit to Switzerland, Belgium, or Luxembourg, where you can still practice your Dirty French in peace. In these countries, notably Switzerland and Luxembourg, the coldness the natives show to all foreigners, black or white, is equal.

pétasse, f
stupid girl, tart, slut
Un groupe de pétasses vient de s'asseoir au bar.
A bunch of bitches just sat down at the bar.

soirée mousse, f
bath night, lit. foam night
Notre disco préférée organise une soirée mousse.
Our favorite disco is having a foam party..

paradis des dragueurs, m
pick-up paradise, lit. heaven of flirtation
La disco c'est aussi le paradis des dragueurs.
The club is also a pick-up paradise.

boîte, f
club, lit. box
Nous sortons en boîte tous les samedis.
We go to clubs every Saturday.

zic, f
music, abbr. of musique
**Cédric danse sur n'importe quelle zic. Il adore se don-
ner en spectacle.**
Cédric dances to any kind of music. He loves to make a scene.

toile, f
movie, lit. canvas
**Loana m'a donné rendez-vous pour aller se faire une
toile.**
Loana gave me an appointment to go and watch a movie.

ciné, m / cinoche, m
movie theater, abbr. of cinéma / with the -oche suffix
J'te paie l'entrée du cinoche.
I'll buy your ticket at the movie theater.

téloche, f / TV, f, / télé, f
television, TV, abbr. of télévision with the -oche suffix
Justin préfère rester chez lui devant la téloche.
Justin prefers to stay home and watch TV.

Time to Leave
mettre les bouts / bouts voiles
to leave, lit. to put the ends / sails
Après cinq ans de mariage, mon mari a mis les voiles.
After five years of marriage, my husband left.

prendre le large

to quit, to go (far) away, lit. to take the large

J'ai envie de prendre le large, pas toi?

I want to go far away, what about you?

lever l'ancre

to leave, lit. to lift the anchor

D'un regard Sarah a compris que son mec voulait lever l'ancre.

In a single look, Sarah understood that her boyfriend wanted to take off.

changer de crèmerie

to change place, lit. to change creamery

Ce bar est trop enfumé. Nous changeons de crèmerie bientôt?

This bar is too smoky. Are we changing places soon?

se faire la malle

to leave, lit. to make the trunk/suitcase

Cette boum est zéro. On se fait la malle discrètement.

This party is a flop. Let's leave discreetly.

bouger

to change place, to leave

Tu bouges pas d'ici, compris?

You're not leaving here, understand?

ficher / foutre le camp

to get out, lit. to put the camp

Fous le camp—j'veux plus te voir!

Get out of here—I don't want to see you any more!

se tailler

to leave, lit. to carve oneself

Putain, il y a le karaoké. C'est le moment de se tailler de ce pub!

F**k, there's karaoke. It's time to leave this pub!

rentrer au bercail

to go back home; bercail means house

Après un trekking de cinq mois en Asie, on était content de rentrer au bercail.

After five months trekking in Asia, we were happy to come back home.

se pieuter

to go to bed, from pieu, wooden stick and slang for bed

Mon grand-père se pieute toujours en laissant la téloche allumée.

My grandfather always goes to bed leaving the TV on.

pioncer

to sleep, again from pieu

Fais pas de bruit, tout le monde pionce.

Don't make noise; everybody's sleeping.

pioncer chez qqn

to sleep over, to crash

J'ai loupé mon dernier bus—j'peux pioncer chez toi?

I missed my last bus—can I crash at your place?

faire la grasse matinée

to sleep in, lit. to make a fat morning

Dimanche, je fais la grasse matinée.

On Sunday, I can sleep in.

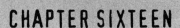

CHAPTER SIXTEEN

La belle et la bête: s/he's Got the Look

If you believe that the French are the most fashionable people in the world, you may have seen too many *haute couture* runway collections on your favorite fashion channel. Paris is considered the fashion capital of the world and French designers create and inspire trends worldwide. Reality, however, will certainly disappoint you. Just as you don't eat *escargots* every day, you won't see an average Joe wearing a *tailleur, a robe de cocktail,* or other *bijoux de la haute couture*, high fashion gems in the streets.

Looks may not be everything in France but they're important nonetheless. French women seem to age gracefully, looking chic at all ages. French men aren't far behind (at least not the *Parisiens*). No matter what their style, the French love to show off their looks. Dressed in jeans and a designer T-shirt or dreadlocked in reggae gear, keeping a specific look is very important. The way you look is who you are, whatever that look may be. While they recognize it's unfair to discriminate against someone based on physical features, the French will do the same based on someone's dress. After all, one doesn't choose his face, but his clothing, yes!

The Look

se mettre sur son 31
to be dressed to the nines, lit. to put oneself on one's 31 (3
piece suit)
**Tu t'es mis sur ton 31 ce matin. T'as quelque chose de
spécial aujourd'hui?**
*You're dressed to the nines this morning. Do you have some-
thing special today?*

flambant neuf
brand-new, lit. burning new
John a acheté un smoking flambant neuf.
John bought a brand-new suit.

être tendance
to be trendy
C'est tendance de porter une jupe sur un jeans.
It's trendy to wear a skirt over jeans.

être dans le vent / dans le coup
to be trendy, lit. to be in the wind / in the hit
Si tu veux être dans le coup, faut changer ton look.
If you want to be trendy, you have to change your look.

ringard, ringarde
out of fashion
Le slip kangourou, c'est super ringard.
Briefs are really out of fashion.

UNDRESSING THE FRENCH

For most French, there's no shopping in a *boutique de haute couture* but in department stores instead. People tend to pay attention to their look and still pay a lot for brand names or fakes. As in the US, jeans are very fashionable and Levis is a popular brand for all generations. Hip-hop clothing is trendy among young people and so is the techno look. Another thing: people don't buy *vêtements* or *habits* in a *magasin d'habillement*. The times and terms have changed: the French will buy *des froques, des fringues, des nippes,* or *des frusques* (all terms previously referring to old or bad-quality clothes) in *un magasin de fringues,* a clothing shop, or *aux nippes*, a second-hand shop. *Se fringuer, se nipper, se saper* mean to dress, while *se dénipper* and *se défroquer* mean to undress.

Once *le falzar, le froc, le fut,* or *le futal*, the pants, are off and after *avoir fait tomber*, taken off, *le top, le sweatshirt, le T-shirt,* and *le pull-over,* you'll discover the underwear. Now you can see *le soutif*, the bra, *le string*, the G-string, *la petite culotte* or in case of a man *le calecif, le calbutte, le calbar,* based on the word *caleçon, le slip kangourou,* the kangaroo brief named after the pocket, or *le slibard* for *le slip* or you'll find a *boxer.*

fringues, fpl

clothes, lit. old bad-quality clothes
Elles sont trop tendance tes frinques.
Your clothes are so trendy.

soutif, m
bra, from soutien-gorge
Allez, Barbara, fais tomber ce soutif!
Come on, Barbara, take that bra off!

Studies show that Americans buy an average of twelve pairs of underwear per year but the French purchase only 2.7 pairs per year. Is it because they wear them inside out too, or because they simply have good cologne and perfume? We'll never know . . .

pébroc, pépin, m
umbrella, from Pépin, an eighth-century French king who
    received a jeweled umbrella from the Pope
Il flotte et j'ai pas de pébroc.
It's raining and I don't have an umbrella.

pompes, fpl
shoes, from pomper, to pump
J'trouve pas mes pompes!
I can't find my shoes!

Shoes are known as *les pompes; les écrase-merde*, the shit steppers; and *les bateaux. Godasses* and *grolles* come from a certain M. Godillot, who invented a special boot for the army. *Cirer les pompes* means 'to wax the shoes' as well as 'to flatter.'

toquante, tocante, f

watch, onomatopoeia, toc sound made by the seconds hand.

Ma toquante indique midi.

My watch says it's noon.

Anatomy

The head, more or less filled, has been compared to different items including *le carafon*, the pitcher, and *la Sorbonne*. The container inspired *la citrouille*, *la caboche*, from *bosse*, bump, *le ciboulot* from *ciboule*, onion, *la boule*, ball, and *le caillou*, the stone.

La cafetière, the coffee percolator, and *le plafond*, the ceiling, maintain the place of the brain, on top.

citrouille, f

nut, lit. pumpkin

T'as rien dans la citrouille.

You've nothing in the nut.

bouille, f

face, from bouillote, hot-water bottle

J'aime pas ta bouille.

I don't like your face.

mirette, f / quinquet, m

eye, from Latin mirare, to look / quinquet from a special lamp

Ouvre tes quinquets!

Open your eyes!

tarin, m, pif, m

nose, from a bird with a pointed nose

T'as un gros pif.

You've got a big nose.

esgourdes, fpl

ears, from old French

Ouvre bien tes esgourdes, je l'dirai pas deux fois.

Listen well; I won't say it twice.

To say someone is hard of hearing, the French use *avoir les portugaises ensablées*, lit. to have sand in the Portuguese, and *être dur de la feuille*, lit. to be hard of the leaf. *Avoir les oreilles en feuilles de chou* applies for dudes with Dumbo ears.

babines, fpl

lips

J'me lèche les babines.

I'm licking my lips.

quenotte, f

tooth, from the Norman quenne, tooth

Kevin devrait se brosser les quenottes plus souvent.

Kevin should brush his teeth more often.

The low Latin word for mouth was *gola*, which has evolved into *la gueule*. It's Dirty French for an animal's mouth and slang for a person's face or mouth. Dirty French also says someone is handsome or pretty if he/she has *une belle gueule*, or *une gueule d'amour*. *Avoir une sale gueule*, lit. to have a dirty face, means ugly. *Le bec*, the beak, is used to mean kiss, and in the realm of food, *becqueter* means to eat.

patte, f
leg or hand, lit. paw
Bas les pattes, c'est à moi!
Hands off, that's mine.

The hand is also called *la paluche* or *la pince*, the claw; hence the expression *se serrer la pince / se serrer les paluches*, to shake hands.

---

guibole, f
leg, from the Norman guibon, leg
Regarde cette paire de guiboles. On voit que Dirk fait du vélo chaque jour.
Look at that pair of legs. You can see that Dirk rides his bike every day.

PRENDRE SON PIED

If you don't pay attention you may step on your partner's feet while dancing. The aggression will be followed by *"Tu m'écrases les petons,"* "You're smashing my little feet," *Tu peux pas regarder où tu mets tes panards,"* "Can't you look where you put your f**king feet?" But don't think you've walked on a dessert or a paintbrush when told: *"Tu viens de m'écraser les nougats / les pinceaux."* Once again, it means that you are a bad dancer and just crushed your partner's feet for a second time. As a good dancer is known to be a good f**k, watch what you're doing and read on.

palpitant, m

heart, lit. that palpites

J'ai le palpitant qui s'emballe en écoutant ta voix sexy.

My heart goes crazy when listening to your sexy voice.

Physical Qualities and Defects

faire de la muscul' / de la gonflette

to do bodybuilding, abbr. of musculation / from gonfler, to inflate

Tristan a fait de la gonflette pendant des années.

Tristan did bodybuilding for years.

abdos, mpl

abs, abbr. of abdominaux

Ken a des abdos de rêve.

Ken has dream abs.

biscoto, m

muscles, from biceps, bicep

Arnold s'est sculpté de gros biscotos.

Arnold has built up big biceps.

plaque de chocolat, f

six-pack, lit. chocolate bar

Y a rien de plus sexy qu'un mec avec une plaque de chocolat et des fesses fermes.

There's nothing sexier than a man with a six-pack and a firm butt.

poignées d'amour, fpl

love handles

Dominique retenait Armand par les poignées d'amour.

Dominique held Armand by his love handles.

bide à bière, m

beer belly

Depuis qu'il a arrêté le sport, Nicolas a chopé un bide à bière.

Since he stopped doing sports, Nicolas has gotten a beer belly.

boudin, m

dog, lit. blood sausage

Ma cousine? Quel boudin!

My cousin? She's a dog!

boudiné, boudinée

stuffed, from boudin

T'es boudinée dans ces jeans.

You're stuffed into those jeans.

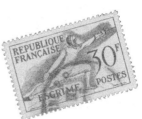

baleine, f

whale

Andréa pèse environ 140 kg et ne comprend pas pourquoi on la surnomme 'la baleine'.

Andréa weighs around 300 pounds and doesn't understand why we've nicknamed her 'the whale.'

canon, m

real peach, lit. cannon

La remplaçante du prof est canon. Je peux même pas me concentrer sur le cours!

The substitute teacher is a real peach. I can't even concentrate on the lesson!

bombe, f

hottie, lit. bomb

Tu t'souviens de la bombe d'hier soir?

Do you remember the hottie from last night?

plante, f

chick, lit. plant

Il est moche mais il sort qu'avec les plus belles plantes.

He's ugly but he goes out with only the cutest chicks.

bien roulée

shapely, lit. well rolled

**La fille du boulanger est trop bien roulée. Je lui touch-
    erai bien les miches.**

*The baker's daughter is very shapely. I'd love to touch her tits
    / butt cheeks.*

bonne

sexy, lit. good, only for women

**Susanne est vraiment trop bonne. Je rêve d'elle toutes
    les nuits.**

Susanne is really too sexy. I dream about her every night.

cradingue

dirty, from crade

Il vit dans un appart cradingue.

He leaves in a dirty flat.

moche, cheumo in verlan

ugly

Avec ses habits démodés, ton frère est trop moche!

With his outdated clothes, your brother is really too ugly!

mocheté, f

dog, lit. ugliness

Cette mocheté de Carole me suit partout depuis deux semaines. Va falloir que ça cesse.

That dog of Carole's has been following me everywhere for two weeks. It has to stop.

laideron, m

dog, from laide, ugly

Le videur lui a dit texto: « Toi, le laideron, tu restes dehors! »

The bouncer told her exactly this: "You, dog, you stay outside!"

Laideron is used for ugly women; it comes from *laide* but the suffix adds an uglier touch. The use of the masculine article reinforces the lack of *féminité,* of the poor woman in question.

cageot, m

ugly person, lit. box

Quel cageot, la fille que Thomas a épousé!

The girl that Thomas married is so ugly!

thon, m

dog, lit. tuna fish

Ta copine est plus que moche—c'est un thon.

Your girlfriend is beyond ugly—she's a dog.

asperge, f

string bean, lit. stalk of asparagus

La plupart des présidents français étaient des asperges, seul l'actuel est une demi-portion.

Most French presidents were string beans, only the current one is a puny runt.

perche, f

twig, lit. pole

La perche s'est tapée la tête dans l'encadrement de la porte. Je lui avais pourtant dit de faire attention!

The twig hit her head against the door frame. And I had told her to be careful!

obus, m

tit, lit. shell (military)

En été, sur les plages de Normandie, des milliers de paires d'obus se dorant au soleil, célèbrent à leur façon le jour-J.

In the summer on the beaches of Normandy, thousands of tits sunbathing celebrate D-day in their own way.

miches, fpl

tits, lit. loaves (of bread)

Elle s'est payée une nouvelle paire de miches avant de partir en vacances à Hollywood.

She bought herself a new pair of tits before going on vacation to Hollywood.

CHAPTER SEVENTEEN

La belle et la bête II:
Looks Aren't Everything

As you may notice, especially when watching a French movie, looks aren't everything. While beauty is valued, attractiveness won't make or break a person. If they're well put together and stylish, it doesn't matter if, in all honesty, they'd look better with a bag over their heads. Take a look at famous French actors like Gérard Dépardieu or Jean Reno. These men won't pass for supermodels, yet they are handsome in their own way, sexy, and extremely talented. Yes, the same goes for women. For every classic French *beauté* like Catherine Deneuve and Brigitte Bardot, there is a sleepy-eyed hottie like Julie Delpy who may not be a bimbo with a giant *paire de seins*, but still gets starring roles.

Does this mean the French are less superficial than Americans are? Not exactly. A *fortune* is spent on clothes, shoes, and beauty products in France. Even ghetto dwellers will save (or steal!) for those new Nikes or a Louis Vuitton *sac à main*.. French women spend more money on face creams and slimming potions than any other women in the world. Just look at the names of makeup lines: L'Oréal, Clinique, Lancôme . . . all French!

Qualités, caractère, qualificatif

avoir un balai dans le cul

to have a stick up one's ass, lit. to have a broom in the ass

Je me demande si un jour Amélie va enlever le balai qu'elle a dans le cul et sourire à la vie.

I wonder if one day Amélie will take out the stick up her ass and enjoy life.

avoir un cœur de pierre

to have a heart of stone

Parle pas d'amour à Bernard; il connaît même pas c'mot. Il a un cœur de pierre.

Don't talk to Bernard about love; he doesn't even know the word. He has a heart of stone.

snober qqn

to not give a shit about someone

Depuis qu'il a gagné à la loterie, Mathieu snobe tous ses anciens amis.

Since winning the lottery Mathieu has snubbed his old friends.

Snob is short for the Latin *sine nobiltas*, 'without nobility.' This derogatory name was used to mark the difference between burghers who were loaded and acted like nobles but lacked noble lineage, and the true noble families. Now *snob* and *snobinard* are derogatory and associated with loaded people who may or may not be noble.

couche-tôt, m

early bird

Ses grands-parents sont des couche-tôt.

His grandparents are early birds.

cafteur, m

tattletale, from cafter, to denounce

Quelle cafteuse Julie. Elle m'avait promis de ne pas te dire ce que j'ai fait!

Julie is such a tattletale. She promised she wouldn't tell you what I did!

mouchard, m

spy, lit. fly, from moucharder

Sale mouchard! T'étonnes pas si plus personne te cause.

Dirty spy! Don't be surprised if nobody talks to you anymore.

tombe, f

someone who is able to keep a secret, lit. grave

Dis lui tout ce que tu veux, il le répètera pas. Pierre est une vraie tombe.

Tell him anything you want, he won't repeat it. Pierre can keep a secret.

poltron, m

wimp

Quel poltron! Il a pas le courage de me dire en face ce qu'il raconte dans mon dos.

What a wimp! He doesn't have the courage to say to my face what he tells behind my back.

demi-portion, f

puny runt, lit. half portion

Tu fais pas le poids contre moi, demi-portion!

You can't compete with me, you puny runt!

mou, molle

wimpy, lit. soft

Le nouveau prof de français est mou.

The new French teacher is a bit wimpy.

se faire marcher dessus

to let people walk all over you

Margot, arrête de t'faire marcher dessus!

Margot, stop letting people walk all over you!

se tenir à carreau

to keep quiet, lit. to keep oneself in a square

Il se tient à carreau depuis que j'lui ai parlé en privé.

He's kept quiet since I spoke to him in private.

faire la gueule à qqn

to be mad at someone, lit. to make the mutt

Je peux savoir au moins pourquoi tu me fais la gueule?

Can I at least know why you're mad at me?

pleurnicher

to whine, from pleurer, to cry

**Cesse de pleurnicher. Une copine de perdue, dix de
     retrouvées !**

Stop whining. Lose one girlfriend and you'll find ten others.

se gaffer, faire gaffe

to be careful

Elle fait gaffe à ne pas blesser les gens.

She's careful not to hurt people's feelings.

s'emmerder

to get bored, lit. to put oneself in the shit

Y a rien à foutre dans ce camping. On s'emmerde grave.

There's nothing to do at this campsite. We're really bored.

avoir le moral à zéro / au fond des baskets

to be down, lit. to have one's morale at zero / in the sneakers

Il a le moral à zéro à cause de ce que tu lui as dit.

He's down because of what you told him.

poule mouillée, f

chicken, lit. wet chicken

J'ai dit à Carole qu'on allait régler ça dehors après les cours. Elle est pas venue cette poule mouillée.

I told Carole we'd settle this outside after class. She didn't show up, that chicken.

lèche-botte / -cul, m, f

bootlicker / asskisser, lit. lick-ass

Ce lèche-cul croit obtenir une promotion comme ça?

This asskisser thinks he will obtain a promotion like that?

pantouflard, pantouflarde

homebody, lit. a guy who stays in his slippers most of the time

Mathias s'est transformé en pantouflard depuis son mariage.

Since his wedding, Mathias has become a homebody.

être le dindon de la farce, m

to be made a fool of, lit. to be the turkey of the joke

**Hilary était le dindon de la farce pendant le dîner de la
compagnie.**

At the company dinner, Hilary was made a fool of.

déconner

to fool around, to bullshit, lit. to pull out (during sex)

**Arrêtons de déconner maintenant. Nous avons du tra-
vail qui nous attend.**

Let's stop fooling around now. We have work waiting for us.

déconneur, déconneuse

bullshitter, lit. someone who pulls out during sex

**Grégoire est un beau déconneur. Il m'a dit que ses par-
ents étaient friqués, mais je viens de savoir qu'il a
grandi avec l'aide sociale!**

*Grégoire is a real bullshitter. He told me his parents are
loaded, but I just found out he grew up on welfare!*

salopard, m

dickhead, from sale, dirty

**Ton ami est un salopard. Il m'a promis du boulot et il l'a
donné à quelqu'un d'autre.**

*Your friend is a dickhead. He promised me a job and he gave it
to somebody else.*

salaud

f**ker, from sale, dirty

Quelle espèce de salaud, mon frère.

My brother is a real f**ker.

être gonflé

to be full of oneself, lit. to be inflated

Je viens d'engager Sylvie et elle me demande déjà une augmentation. Elle est gonflée la nana!

I just hired Sylvie and she's already asked me for a raise. She's pretty full of herself!

racaille, f

scum

Traiter de racaille la jeunesse des banlieues a été la raison des violentes émeutes de 2005 en France.

Calling the youth of the suburbs scum was the reason behind the violent 2005 riots in France.

fêtard, m

partier

Tous les soirs en disco, j'suis un fêtard, et alors?

At the disco every night, I'm a partier; so what?

foireur, m

partier, from foire, fair

Quelle foireuse! Céline veut sortir s'amuser toute la nuit.

What a partier! Céline wants to go out and have fun all night long.

chic type, m

nice guy

Les parents de Laura adorent le nouveau copain de leur fille. Ils sont sûrs qu'il s'agit d'un chic type.

Laura's parents adore their daughter's new boyfriend. They're sure he's a nice guy.

couche-tard, m

night owl, lit. person who goes to bed late

Quelle couche-tard ma femme. Tous les soirs la lumière reste allumée jusqu'à deux heures du matin parce que madame veut lire ses livres . . .

My wife is such a night owl. Every night the light stays on until 2 in the morning because she wants to read her books . . .

rouleur de mécaniques, m

show-off, lit. mechanical roller

Michael donne l'impression d'avoir beaucoup de succès, mais j'sais qu'il n'est qu'un rouleur de mécaniques.

Michael gives the impression that he is really successful, but I know he's just a show-off.

mettre qqn hors de soi

to get on someone's nerves, lit. to put someone out of himself

Mon colocataire me met hors de moi, en écoutant sa musique hip hop à 7 h!

My neighbor gets on my nerves, playing his hip-hop music at 7 am!

ne pas avoir froid aux yeux

to have the nerve to do something, lit. to not have cold eyes

Jean a vraiment pas froid aux yeux pour venir chez moi me dire ces horreurs!

Jean has got some nerve to come to my house and tell me these awful things!

avoir une sacrée paire de couilles

to have some balls, lit. have a sacred pair of balls

T'as vraiment une sacrée paire de couilles pour te pointer comme ça au bureau après quatre semaines d'absence!

You've got some balls to come to work as if nothing happened after a four-week absence!

balaise

strong

Samantha cherche deux types balaises pour déménager.

Samantha is looking for two strong guys to help her move.

or

good at something

Denis est balaise en gymnastique.

Denis is very good at gymnastics.

or

difficult, hard

L'examen de maths était vachement balaise.

The math exam was very hard.

traiter qqn comme de la merde

to treat someone like shit

Traite pas ta sœur comme de la merde!

Don't treat your little sister like shit!

vicelard, m

kinky person

Les Allemands sont des vicelards. Toute personne qui a vu un porno allemand le sait.

Germans are kinky. Anyone who has ever watched German porn knows that.

avoir du bol / du cul / du pot
to have much luck, lit. to have bowl/ass/pot
Marilyn joue au poker et elle a toujours du cul.
Marilyn plays poker and is always very lucky.

The French claim that one is either lucky when gambling or lucky in love. In the expression *avoir un bol de cocu*, lit. to have a bowl of 'cheated on,' *le bol de cocu* indicates that to be lucky, the person has to be cheated by his/her partner.

se débiner
to escape from one's duties
Oscar trouve toujours un prétexte pour se débiner de ses responsabilités.
Oscar always finds a way to escape from his duties.

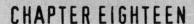

CHAPTER EIGHTEEN

Amour toujours:
Love Is a Wonderful Thing

The French have a reputation as the world's best lovers. This title is something they are extremely proud of, and most French people will happily go out of their way to prove it to you. But it is not their lovemaking skills that place the French on this pedestal. It's everything else—the heartfelt initial conversations, the romantic gestures of giving flowers and writing love letters and sweet poetry. It has nothing to do with the whiny complaints of Alphonse de Lamartine, or the sweet verses of *le poète des roses*, Pierre de Ronsard.

You'll adore the cute nicknames lovers give each other, ranging from vegetables to flowers and everything in between. They say *L'amour a ses raisons que la raison ne connaît pas*, that love has reasons that reason doesn't know. In this spirit, you can call your mate every possible name in the book without looking like a jerk. Even normally insulting words said sweetly will charm most French. Would you mind if your *chéri* called you a dog or a rat? In France it will win you big points.

You can nickname an enemy easily and you can call a child *mon petit bonhomme* without problems, but to nickname someone you really care about implies that some intimacy has already been shared. You wouldn't like to be called sweetie, angel, or honey by a person you had just met, as it would be meaningless. The French believe that nicknames are the expression of complicity and strength between two people.

But in order to make the most out of your trip to France and the opposite (or same!) sex, we have to put a few rules down first. Inviting or accepting an invitation to dinner doesn't necessarily mean sex afterward. A cozy restaurant is more romantic than a crowded pub or noisy disco. The third date rule doesn't hold in France, and the common first-date kiss is definitely not *de rigueur*. As for dinner, your date may just be hungry and want to get to know you better. So don't be upset if s/he doesn't follow you to your room afterward or recoils from a kiss; it's just a cultural difference.

Love at First Sight

kiffer
to like, from the Arabic
Roméo kiffait trop Juliette qu'il en est mort pour elle.
Romeo loved Juliette so much that he died for her.

B.C.B.G.
good-looking and well-mannered, lit. bon chic, bon genre
Tout parent veut un gendre B.C.B.G.
*Every parent desires a good-looking and well-mannered
    son-in-law.*
Or
Barbie, abbr. of Beau Cul Belle Gueule, lit. nice ass, nice face
Samuel ne cherche qu'une femme B.C.B.G.
Samuel wants a Barbie and nothing else.

gueule d'amour, m

cute guy, lit. love face

La gueule d'amour du pub nous a invitées à diner.

The cute guy from the pub invited us to dinner.

faire / lancer un clin d'œil à qqn

to wink at someone, lit. to do/throw a wink

Une bonnasse lui a lancé un clin d'oeil, et il est déjà amoureux.

A hottie winked at him, and he is already in love with her.

coup de foudre, m

love at first sight, lit. bolt of lightning

Juliette croyait pas au coup de foudre, jusqu'à ce qu'elle rencontre Roméo.

Juliette didn't believe in love at first sight until she met Romeo.

taper dans l'œil de qqn

to catch someone's eye, lit. to punch someone in the eye

Evan m'a tout de suite tapé dans l'œil.

Evan immediately caught my eye.

avoir le béguin pour qqn

to have a crush on somebody, from béguin, little hat

Rodrigo ne l'avouera jamais, mais il a le béguin pour toi.

Rodrigo will never admit it, but he has a crush on you.

faire craquer qqn

to fall for someone

Tu me fais craquer, tu sais . . .

I'm falling for you, you know . . .

craquer pour qqn

to not resist someone, lit. to crack for someone

Léa a craqué pour un instructeur de plongée.

Léa fell for a scuba diving instructor.

être fou de qqn / qqch

to be crazy about someone / something

Je suis fou de gros culs—J-Lo et Beyoncé sont les femmes de mes rêves.

I'm crazy about big butts—J-Lo and Beyoncé are my dream women.

Seduction

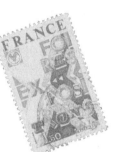

allumeur, allumeuse

teaser

Quelle allumeuse, Naomi!

Naomi is such a tease!

allumer

to tease, lit. to light

Nicole allume tous les beaux gosses qu'elle voit.

Nicole teases every cute guy she sees.

flirt, m

flirtation

C'est pas sérieux entre nous, c'est juste un flirt de plus.

It isn't serious between us, it's just another flirtation.

drague, f

flirtation, from draguer, to drag

Prends exemple sur Luca, c'est un as de la drague.

Follow Luca's example; he's a pro at flirting.

dragueur, dragueuse

flirt, lit. dragger

J'te savais pas si dragueur.

I didn't know you were such a flirt.

baratin, m

chatter

**Faut pas écouter tout ce qu'elles disent, c'est que du
baratin.**

Don't listen to everything they say, it's just chatter.

baratiner

to sweet-talk, to chat up

**Arrête de me baratiner, Tom. J'suis pas si désespérée
pour sortir avec toi!**

*Stop sweet-talking me, Tom. I'm not desperate enough to go
out with you!*

baratineur, baratineuse

smooth talker

**Simon est un grand baratineur. Écoute toutes les con-
neries qu'il raconte pour séduire les minettes.**

*Simon is such a smooth talker. Listen to all the bullshit he
says to seduce chicks.*

faire du pied / genou

to play footsie, lit. to make foot / knee

**À la fete de Noël l'année passée, j'ai fait du pied sous
la table à la femme saoule de mon boss.**

*At the Christmas party last year, I played footsie under the
table with my boss's drunken wife.*

faire du gringue

to seduce

Tu serais pas en train de me faire du gringue par hasard?

You wouldn't be trying to seduce me by any chance?

Faire du gringue probably comes from *grignon*, bread
used by fishermen to *appâter le poisson,* attract the fish.
Taquiner le poisson, lit. to tease the fish, is also used in
the same way, meaning to see if there may be some positive outcome.

avoir une touche / ouverture

to have a chance, lit. to have a touch/opening

**Valentin avait une touche avec Betty mais il n'a pas
voulu aller plus loin.**

Valentin had a chance with Betty but had no desire to go further.

courir après qqn

to chase someone

**Joey a couru après Barbara pendant des années avant
qu'elle accepte de sortir avec lui.**

*Joey had been chasing Barbara for years before she agreed to
go out with him.*

avoir / donner un rencard

to have/make a date

J'peux pas rester; j'ai un rencard.

I can't stay; I've got a date.

(se) dégoter une fille / un mec
to find, lit. to dig up
Tu l'as dégoté où ton mec?
Where did you find your boyfriend?

FRENCH TOUCH

When intimate, French partners call each other all kinds of sweet, strange, and unexpected names. Those uncreative souls will use the most common sweet nicknames like *mon amour*, (my) love, *mon coeur*, my heart, *ma douce*, my sweet, *ma belle* or *mignon*, cutie. Adjectives referring to appearance are good too: *mon petit, ma petiote, mon grand, mon p'tit grassouillet*, my fatty one. Even intelligence can be put in question: *mon petit crétin, ma petite idiote*. The trick is to use an adjective that balances the negative aspect of the noun.

Animals are an important *source d'inspiration*. Cute little bugs are common, as in *ma coccinelle*, my ladybug, *ma puce, pupuce*, my flea. Other animal names include *chaton, minet*, cat, *poussin*, chicken, *mon loulou*, my wolf, and so on; while religion motivates *mon p'tit diable*, and *mon ange*, my angel. The vegetable world reigns with *mon chou, mon chouchou*, and *mon sucre*. And everything becomes sweeter when followed by *en sucre*, of sugar, or *d'amour*, of love: *mon lapin en sucre* and *mon lapin d'amour*.

Beginner's Luck

voir la vie en rose
to see life through rose-colored glasses, lit. to see life in pink
Elle m'énerve avec sa manie de voir la vie en rose.
She's getting on my nerves with the way she sees life through rose-colored glasses.

être sur un petit nuage
to be on cloud nine, lit. to be on a little cloud
Les jeunes couples sont sur un petit nuage, et après vient l'orage.
Young couples are often on cloud nine and then comes the storm.

balcon, m
tits, lit. balcony
Y a du monde au balcon!
She has big boobs.

The literal translation of *y a du monde au balcon* is, there are a lot of people on the balcony. This expression implies a woman's *décolleté* is very generous and that the woman wears a bra; otherwise there would be no balcony to hold up the breasts!

bichonner
to spoil, to take great care of someone/something
J'vais te bichonner chéri.
I'm going to spoil you, baby.

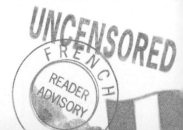

câlin, m (and adjective)

cuddle, cuddly or tender

Nos amis arrêtent pas de s'faire des câlins quand on sort en couples.

Our friends can't stop cuddling each other when we double-date.

PAR TOUS LES SEINS

All kinds of words come to mind when you are thinking breasts. Some have many 'o's and remind us of their soft and round form, *le roploplo* and *le lolo*. The repetition of some phonemes as in *le néné*, and the previous ones, is certainly due to the fact that breasts come in pairs. In French it's common to add *une paire* before the slang word used to refer to them. Big juicy fruits are also a perfect inspiration: *les melons* and the milky *noix de coco*, coconuts. *Le nichon* and *le nibard* come from *nicher* and *nid*, nest; a corset pushing up the breasts to look like two eggs in a nest. Don't forget breasts are tools, and the breastfeeding function of the breasts led to *le téton* from the verb *téter*.

Robert refers to one of the industrial pioneers of baby bottles, *biberons*. A popular brand name in the mid to late 1800s, *le biberon Robert à long tube*, became synonymous with *le biberon* itself. In 1910, the same product was judged risky to babies' health and the producer had to put a *tétine en plastique,* plastic nipple, on top of the bottle. Thanks to a popular advertising and marketing campaign, the brand name *Robert* became synonymous with breast.

câliner

to caress, to cuddle

Pour certaines personnes être câlinées vaut mieux que baiser.

For some people being caressed is better than f**king.

Câlin is one of those words that is sometimes used as a euphemism for sex. One may ask for a *câlin* thinking of sex and feel completely misunderstood or unloved when only cuddled. On the other hand, your partner may think that you're only going to cuddle with him/her and might be unprepared or offended by your overtly sexual advances. *Bisous* is a cute word for kiss but is also a euphemism for blowjob. To avoid disaster, be absolutely sure you and your date share the same definition.

caresser, donner une caresse

to caress, stroke

Après avoir fait l'amour, les femmes aiment être caressées mais les hommes préfèrent aller dormir.

After sex women love to be caressed, but men prefer to go straight to sleep.

suçon, m

kiss mark, love bite, from sucer, to suck

En voyant le suçon sur le cou d'Carlos, sa femme a su qu'il l'avait trompée.

Seeing the hickey on Carlos's neck, his wife knew he had cheated on her.

chatouiller, faire des chatouilles
to tickle
Me chatouille pas trop ou j'vais me pisser parmi.
Don't tickle me too much or I'm going to pee my pants.

Laughing is a mix of pain and pleasure and as such, the power of tickling is not to be underestimated. Don't believe us? Foot tickling was used as a form of torture in the *moyen âge*, Middle Ages. Tickling can also cause strong sexual reactions. As with drugs, it can be poison or medicine depending on the dosage. Don't be shy to use this *technique*, remembering that the proverb "*Femme qui rit, à moitié dans ton lit*," a woman that laughs is halfway to your bed, holds true even today.

Shit Happens

poser un lapin
to stand someone up, lit. to put a rabbit
Félix s'demande pourquoi Kara lui a posé un lapin.
Félix wonders why Kara stood him up.

se prendre une veste / un râteau
to be rejected, lit. to receive a jacket / a rack
James vient de s' prendre une veste.
James has just been rejected.

tromper qqn

to cheat someone

Vanessa a trompé son copain avec un touriste allemand.

Vanessa cheated on her boyfriend with a German tourist.

cocu, m

cuckold (man who is cheated on), from coq, rooster or coucou

Pour se bagarrer dans un pub en France, il suffit de traiter votre voisin de bar de 'cocu'.

To get in a bar fight in France, you only have to call your bar mate a cuckold.

cocufier qqn, faire cocu qqn,

to cheat on someone, from cocu

Sa femme le fait cocu depuis plusieurs mois et il soup-çonne rien.

His wife has been cheating on him for months and he doesn't suspect anything.

Cocu may be an old form of *coucou,* the bird that inspired those hideous Bavarian clocks. This bird is known to put its egg in the nest of another species in order to avoid parenting responsibilities. Much like today's fathers, only back then there was no Judge Judy to ensure child support payments. This seems to fit the perfect image of one's wife's lover, for how many men having affairs with married women would step up to the plate if they got pregnant? The term *cocu* is nowadays attributed to the cheated person in the couple, be it male or female.

étouffer
to suffocate, lit. to choke
J'étouffe avec toi, laisse-moi vivre!
I'm suffocating with you, let me breathe!
Lit. I'm choking with you, let me live!

faire le point
to think things over, lit. to make the point
Sa femme s'est éloignée pour faire le point.
His wife went away to think things over.

Game Over

plaquer / larguer / lourder qqn
to dump someone, lit. to plate / to drop / send to the door
Tamara a plaqué son mec et veut plus entendre parler de lui.
Tamara dumped her boyfriend and doesn't want to hear about him any more.

envoyer balader / paître qqn
to blow someone off, lit. to take for a walk / to send someone grazing
Patricia m'a envoyé balader quand j'lui ai demandé de sortir avec moi.
Patricia blew me off when I asked her to go out with me.

envoyer pisser / chier
to be sent away, lit. to send someone to pee / shit
Les mecs, faut tous les envoyer pisser.
All men should be sent away.

envoyer péter

to send someone packing, lit. to send to explode

Matthias en avait marre de sa copine et l'a envoyée péter.

Matthias was tired of his girlfriend and sent her packing.

arrêter les frais

to make a clean break, lit. to stop the expenses

Il vaut mieux arrêter les frais—notre histoire est un fiasco.

It's better to make a clean break—our relationship is a fiasco.

tourner la page

to turn the page

Y a deux ans que Jerry et Jeanne se sont quittés mais il veut pas tourner la page.

Jerry and Jeanne split two years ago but he doesn't want to turn the page.

New Game

se remettre ensemble

to get back together, lit. to put each other together again

Remettons nous ensemble. J'vais changer—j'te promets.

Let's get back together. I'll change—I promise!

recoller les morceaux

to get back together, lit. to glue the pieces back together

Donne-nous une seconde chance. On peut recoller les morceaux.

Give us a second chance. We can get back together.

CHAPTER NINETEEN

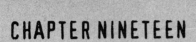

Voulez-vous coucher avec moi ce soir?:

Partners and Their Private Parts

French cultural tradition is stronger than their republican triad, *liberté, égalité, fraternité*. It seems the French afford men some leeway to chase, as if it were in their blood or there was a genetic weakness involved. For a woman, however, only derogatory terms apply. While a man who frequents many women is simply known as a *coureur de jupons*, skirt chaser, a woman who goes out with many men is called *une pute*, whore. On the other hand, women who are difficult to conquer are also verbal targets—a classic case of damned if they do, damned if they don't.

Homosexual slang varies with the times. *La (grande) folle*, the queer, lit. the (big) crazy woman, was popularized by the French-Italian movie *La Cage aux Folles*, the birdcage, or more correctly, the cage of queens (1978), with Michel Serrault. The movie offers a humorous vision of effeminate men, dressing, speaking, and acting like women. After a lifetime of thirty years, the term *la (grande) folle* is no longer in use. Nowadays, *homo* and *gay* are the most common slang terms, but in third place is *PD*. *PD, or pédé*, is the abbreviation of *pédéraste*, from the ancient Greek model of homosexuality—men with teenagers. It also gave birth to *la pédale*, also popularized in a movie: *Pédale Douce*, sweet gay, or lit. soft pedal. The word *la tapette*, gay, lit. little hit / kick, shows another stereotype of homosexual men—their supposed lack of strength and masculinity. In this same genre are *tante* and *tantouze*, auntie, which suggest feminine qualities.

Lesbians are sometimes called *gouines*, from *gouin*, cad, and *broute-gazon*, carpet-muncher, popularized by the film *Gazon maudit* (1995) by Josiane Balasko. While *gazon maudit* translates literally as 'evil pubic triangle,' the tame English version was retitled *French Twist*. Still, you'll most often hear *lesbienne* or *gay*.

coincé/e du bulbe
uptight, lit. having one's bulb stuck
Catherine est vachement coincée du bulbe; impossible de plaisanter avec elle.
Catherine is really uptight; it's impossible to joke around with her.

sainte nitouche, f
goody two-shoes, lit. a saint that doesn't touch
Arrête de jouer la sainte nitouche. On sait que t'as couché avec Sébastien hier soir. Il nous a tout dit.
Stop the goody two-shoes act. We know you slept with Sébastien last night. He told us everything.

être en manque (de sexe)
to be sex starved, to not get any
Benoît, tu dois être en manque pour fantasmer sur elle.
Benoît, you must be sex starved to fantasize about her.

baisable

f**kable, from baiser to f**k

Sarah est baisable mais j'en voudrais pas comme copine.

Sarah's f**kable but not girlfriend material.

baiseur, baiseuse

f**k

Lara est une sacrée bonne baiseuse.

Lara is a really good f**k.

mal baisé, mal baisée

sexually unsatisfied, lit. badly f**ked

Steve a tout de suite su que Julie était mal baisée.

Steve knew right away that Julie was sexually unsatisfied.

bon / mauvais au pieu

good / bad in bed, lit. good in the stake

Denise est bonne au pieu, mais j'pourrais pas vivre avec elle.

Denise is good in bed, but I couldn't live with her.

bon / mauvais coup, m

good / bad f**k, lit. good / bad hit

T'es un sacré bon coup.

You're a good f**k.

chaud lapin, m

horndog, guy who sleeps around, lit. hot rabbit

Stéphane était un chaud lapin jusqu'à ce qu'il se marie avec Antoinette.

Stéphane used to sleep around until he married Antoinette.

chaud du manche / de la pince, m

horndog, lit. a guy with a hot stick/claw

Ton mec est un chaud du manche.

Your boyfriend's a horndog.

Casanova / Don Juan, m

Casanova

Ne tombe pas amoureuse d'Ismet. C'est qu'un Casanova.

Don't fall in love with Ismet. He's nothing but a Casanova.

enjambeur / tombeur, m

womanizer, lit. one who walks over / makes people fall

Léonard est un infatigable enjambeur.

Léonard is an insatiable womanizer.

coureur de jupons, m

skirt-chaser

Quel coureur de jupons, ton petit frère Mikey!

What a skirt-chaser your little brother Mikey is!

queutard, m

man-whore, from queue, dick

Claude est juste un queutard de merde.

Claude is only a shitty man-whore.

chaudasse, f

hottie, from chaude, hot, with the -asse suffix

Donne un coup d'œil à la chaudasse derrière nous.

Look at the hotties behind us.

garce, f

bitch

Ma coloc', cette garce, a chipé mon homme.

My roommate, that bitch, took my man away from me.

salope, f

bitch, slut, from sale, dirty

Cette salope t'a quitté pour ton meilleur ami!

That bitch left you for your best friend!

belle cochonne, f

dirty slut, lit. cute pig

Toi, t'es une belle cochonne!

You, you're a dirty slut!

chienne en chaleur, f

bitch in heat

Tu t'comportes comme une chienne en chaleur.

You're acting like a bitch in heat.

hangar à bittes, m

slut, whore, lit. dick storage unit

Carmen n'est plus une petite fille innocente, elle est devenue un vrai hangar à bittes.

Carmen isn't an innocent little girl; she's become a real whore.

trainée, f

prostitute, whore, lit. (someone who leaves) a trail

La traînée fait chaque soir des allers-retours devant notre immeuble.

The prostitute walks back and forth in front of our building every night.

crasseuse, f

whore, lit. filthy girl

Ta sœur est une petite crasseuse! Elle s'est tapée tous les gars de la cité.

Your sister is a whore! She's banged every guy in town.

mangeuse d'hommes, f

man-eater

Catherine me fait peur. On m'a dit qu'elle était une mangeuse d'hommes.

Catherine scares me. I was told she's a man-eater.

Minorities

bi

bi

J'ai choisi de ne pas choisir; j'suis bi.

I've chosen not to choose; I'm bi.

travelo, m

tranny, from travesti, transvestite

Ce night est plein de travelos.

That nightclub is filled with trannies.

être de l'autre bord / du bâtiment

to be gay, lit. to be from the other shore/ from the building

Je t'ai jamais vu avec une poulette, tu serais pas de l'autre bord?

I've never seen you with a chick; are you gay?

virer de bord

to change sides/teams

C'est drôle; on pensait tous que tu avais viré de bord.

It's funny; we all thought you'd changed teams.

être PD (pédé) comme un phoque / foc

to be queer as a three dollar bill, lit. to be as gay as a seal/sail

J't'assure cet acteur est pédé comme un phoque.

I assure you, this actor is queer as a three dollar bill.

This strange term, *pédé comme un phoque*, seems not to refer to seals, as we've no reason to assume seals are gay. *Phoque* is pronounced the same as *foc*, a special sail that is pushed by the wind, of course, from behind.

matage, m. noun
checking someone out
Les plages en été, y a pas mieux pour le matage de gonzesses.
Beaches in the summer are the best places for checking out chicks.

mater
to check out, lit. to look at
T'as vu comme elle t'a maté?
Did you see how she checked you out?

se rincer l'oeil
to get an eyeful, lit. to rinse one's eye
Vos voisins doivent bien se rincer l'œil quand vous baisez sur votre terrasse.
Your neighbors must get an eyeful when you f**k on your terrace.

Sex—Parts

à cul nu
naked, lit. with bare ass
Ça m'excite de voir ma femme se promener à cul nu dans la maison.
It excites me to see my wife walking naked around the house.

Usually tabooed and excluded by those with good taste, the ass lives up to its potential in Dirty French. Its paleness (in many cases) leads to the expression *montrer la lune,* lit. to show the moon. The way it seems to dance when looked at from behind gave way to the name *le valseur,* waltzer. *L'avoir dans le baba* or *dans le cul,* to take it in the ass, is normally used to say someone has been duped but is also used to describe sodomy. *Croupe* and *croupion* in French refer to horses and birds' asses and used in Dirty French for humans as well. *Le derche* is a vulgar form of *le derrière,* the behind. The cutesy *le popotin,* with its *o* sounds, indicates a round and soft ass as well as having symmetrical buttocks, *les fesses.*

panier, m
butt, lit. basket
Pablo n'arrête pas de mettre la main au panier.
Pablo won't stop touching my butt.

trou du cul / de balle, m
asshole, lit. hole of the ball
Violette s'est faite défoncer le trou de balle.
XXX: Too Dirty to Translate

rondelle, f
asshole, lit. round, circle
Xavier marche bizarrement car Pierre-Yves lui a pété la rondelle hier soir.
XXX: Too Dirty to Translate

PENIS ENVY

Many Frenchmen refer to their reproductive organs as the precious *bijoux de famille*, or *bourse*, purse. Some do-it-yourselfers may make a comparison with their favorite tools: *le chalumeau*, welding torch, *le piston*, *lance d'arrosage*, hosepipe, or *gaule*, pole. Some looking for a quickie will see *un levier de vitesse*, to do it even faster, while others willing to feed the world will compare it to *une asperge*, *une baguette*, *une carotte*, *une friandise*, delicacy, *un sucre d'orge*, rock candy, *un os à mœlle*, marrow bone....

The conqueror will speak of his *baïonnette*, *bâton de maréchal*, *dague*, or *trique*, or will see an alert *sentinelle* in his pants. *Le dard*, a bee's stinger, is a weapon coming from the animal world and a commonly used slang term for penis. Humorous guys will entertain you and make you laugh with their *guignol*, or *polichinelle*. The big travelers may try to show you their *obélisque de Louxor* or *obélisque de la place Vendôme*. The music buff will seek to make you play some special *musique de chambre* for him by offering you his *fifre*, *pipeau*, *sifflet*, *flûte à un trou*, *flûte à bec*. The sea lover will propose to hang you on his *bitte*, to take *le gouvernail* for a while, or ask you if *le périscope* is out. In any case, *le baigneur* will be more than pleased to go for a swim with you.

Poetry inspires names like *le grand chauve à col roulé*, *la veuve et les orphelines*, *le service-trois-pièces*, *le cigare à moustache*, or *le serpent à un œil*. The arrogant lad will speak about his *membre*, member, *jambe du milieu*, middle leg, or *troisième jambe*. Modesty will push some French to refer to it as *une limace*, slug, or *un bigorneau*, winkle. *Zizi*, *zigounette*, from *zob*, Arabic name for dick, *quéquette*, *robinet, popaul,* Peter, can be seen as signs of immaturity or an attempt to bring back innocence and childhood.

You will certainly be surprised when offered a view of your Frenchman's *pine* and you realize that it doesn't have anything to do with pine, not even the smell. Finally, you'll have a taste of French culture when exposed to *les vals-euses,* a term popularized by a movie of the same name by Bertrand Blier in 1974, starring two excellent actors, Gérard Depardieu and Patrick Dewaere.

les seins / le cul à l'air

bare tits / ass, lit. tits / ass exposed to the air

Sur les plages les Françaises se baladent les seins à l'air.

On the beach, Frenchwomen walk around topless.

bite, bitte, queue, f

cock, lit. bollard / tale

Karim a sorti sa queue du pantalon et l'a frottée contre Louise.

XXX: Too Dirty to Translate

couilles, fpl

balls, from lower Latin colea, testicles

Annette a donné un coup de pied dans les couilles d'un exhibitionniste.

Annette kicked the balls of an exhibitionist.

burnes, fpl

balls, from a French patois

Caresse-lui les burnes, tous les mecs aiment ça.

Caress his balls; all men like that.

gland, m

head of the dick, lit. acorn, knob

Lucy lui a léché le gland avant de le mordiller.

XXX: Too Dirty to Translate

grand chauve à col roulé, m

dick, lit. the big bald with a rolled collar

Karine n'a pas encore vu le grand chauve à col roulé.

Karine hasn't seen a dick yet.

roubignoles, fpl

balls, from a French patois, robin, male goat

Valérie lui a léché les roubignoles.

XXX: Too Dirty to Translate

Pussy

But enough of penis talk; Dirty French has been greatly inspired by the female organs as well. If 'cunt' is a 'bad word' in English, the French prefer positive names for the vagina. They refer to it often as *une chatte* or the *verlan teuch*. The feline gave other words such as *chagatte*, *minou,* and *minette*, pussycat. There's the fun-loving *la salle des fêtes,* while *la moule,* the mussel, reminds us of the shape, smell, or taste. *Foufoune, fouf'* are common for vulva, traditionally used in *Elles se lèchent la foufoune*, they lick each other's pussy. *Baba* means pussy but also means ass. *J'vais te le mettre dans le baba*, I'm going to put it in your pussy (or ass), can lead to severe miscommunication, which in turn may lead to big relationship problems. Last but not least, terms like *clito*, clit, *la praline, le haricot,* or *le bouton d'amour*, the love button, are all nicknames for the clitoris. If you don't know where that one is, put down the book and dial 9-1-1.

touffe, f
bush, lit. tuft
Rase-toi la touffe!
Shave your bush!

bouton d'amour, m
love button
**Monica regardait Jérôme dans les yeux en se titillant
le bouton d'amour.**
XXX: Too Dirty to Translate

Tools

capote (anglaise), f
french letter, condom
T'as pris des capotes avec toi?
Did you bring condoms with you?

préservatif, m
condom, from préserver, to preserve
Sans préservatif, sans moi!
Without a condom, without me!

godemichet, gode, m
dildo
Aude a sorti un gode de dessous son lit et a joué avec.
Aude took out a dildo from under the bed and played with it.

vibro, m
vibrator, abbr. of vibrateur
**Depuis qu'Emilie s'est acheté un vibro, elle a meilleur
mine.**
Since Emilie bought a vibrator, she looks a lot better.

CHAPTER TWENTY

Plan 'Q':
Dirty, Dirtier, and Dirtiest French

As a *connoisseur*, you have surely kept this section for dessert, the *crème brûlée* of Dirty French. If you have chosen to start the book with this section, you're the kind of person who eats dessert first. In any event welcome to the dark side, the dirtiest part of Dirty French. Rather than provide detailed information, Dirty French has a quantity over quality approach—this chapter is one of the longest for a reason.

Are the French all sexual predators? According to US laws, yes. Are they all depraved? Using the same standards, yes again. The age of consent is 15 years old for any kind of sexual relations, whether heterosexual or homosexual. Citizens are free to do what they want with their bodies with no religion setting the legal code. Many *pays* claim to have a separation of church and state, but are still heavily influenced by whichever religion sways the masses. In France, home to Catholics and large Muslim and Jewish minorities, this actually holds true. So don't call the police if you see an old man with a teenager of 15; it's perfectly legal.

Warm Up

bander

to get a hard-on, lit. to tense

Ta voix sexy me fait bander comme un porc.

Your sexy voice gives me a hard-on.

débander

to get soft, opposite of bander

Après avoir pris du Viagra, le gars ne pouvait plus débander.

After the guy took Viagra, he couldn't get soft.

barreau / gourdin, m

hard-on, lit. bar, billy club

J'ai un gourdin dans mon slip.

I've got a hard-on in my underwear.

trique, f

woody, lit. big stick

En regardant sa cousine en bikini à la piscine, Pierrot a eu la trique.

While gazing at his cousin in her bikini at the swimming pool, Pierrot got a woody.

mouiller

to get wet

À peine tu lui touches le cul, elle mouille.

As soon as you touch her butt, she gets wet.

mouille, f

love juice

La mouille coulait de sa chatte le long de ses jambes.

XXX: Too Dirty to Translate

mouillée

wet

Après quelques caresses, Célia est déjà tout mouillée.

After a few caresses, Célia is already wet.

avoir le créateur en larme

to have pre-ejaculate, lit. to have tears on the creator

**Fanny est trop belle. Quand on la voit on a le créateur
en larme.**

Fanny is too cute. When we see her we have pre-ejaculate.

se branler

to masturbate, lit. to shake oneself

Elle m'a dit d'aller me branler ailleurs.

She told me to go masturbate somewhere else.

s'astiquer le manche

to jerk off, lit. to polish one's stick

Il s'astique le manche devant un magazine de cul.

He's jerking off looking at a porno mag.

(se) doigter

to finger (oneself)

Suzanne se doigte souvent dans les chiottes publiques.

XXX: Too Dirty to Translate

To have a date with *Mme Poignet*, Mrs. Wrist, or *la veuve à cinq doigts*, the five-fingered widow, in the country of individualism is quite frequent. If most men do it, they don't openly speak about it. If even half of women do it, they certainly don't speak about it!

branlette, f
jerking off, from branler, to shake
Il préfère la branlette à la baise.
He prefers jerking off to f**king.

first Base

As you may know, the French aren't good at foreign languages in part because they have a hard time rolling the 'r.' To neutralize this defect, they found other things to roll that make people envy them. Can you rouler une pelle, roll a shovel, or roll a skate, rouler un patin? No, but that's what they call a French kiss, though you're more likely to hear them as *le baiser avec la langue, le patin, la pelle*, or *le palot* in France.

rouler une pelle / un palot / un patin à qqn
to French-kiss someone, lit. to roll someone a shovel / ice skate
Il crève d'envie de lui rouler une pelle.
He's dying to French-kiss her.

Second Base

There aren't many expressions in French (or even English for that matter) for Second Base, because once couples move past kissing, the natural next step involves items below the belt, known as Third Base.

peloter
to feel someone up, lit. to pet
Kati a laissé son ami Chris la peloter.
Kati let her boyfriend Chris feel her up.

Third Base

Not quite at Home Base, yet, Third Base is the next best thing. Touching, licking, stroking, sucking, and any other activity below the belt will be found here. Study up to be able to go down in true Dirty French style.

tailler une pipe à qqn
to give a blowjob, lit. to carve someone a pipe
Sandra lui a taillé une pipe au cinéma.
Sandra gave him a blowjob at the movie theater.

More blowjob euphemisms include: *faire un pompier à qqn*, to make a fireman to someone, and *faire une gâterie*, to give a little treat.

Cunnilingus is more widely known as *faire minette, lécher la chatte,* or *le minou,* to lick the pussy, *brouter la chatte,* or *le gazon,* to graze, *descendre à la cave,* to go down to the cellar. A *broute-gazon* is a carpet muncher. In the case of two lesbians, people will use the expression *faire une soudure,* to make a joint. *Bouffer le cul, bouffer la chatte,* and *bouffer la queue* all connect food and sex. We already told you that the French take their cuisine seriously.

branlette espagnole, f

tit-wank, lit. Spanish masturbation

Pascal est sorti avec Dorothée pour les branlettes espagnoles.

Pascal went out with Dorothée for tit-wanks.

This expression draws on the stereotype of large Spanish breasts. Sex acts that bring pleasure to men without the risk of pregnancy and danger of fatherhood are few and far between. One can only assume titty-f**king is an important part of Spanish culture, as their birthrate is currently one of the lowest in Europe.

Home Base

You're here at last! It may be months or just a few days after your first date in France, but your partner is finally ready to take the next step. Now it's decision time: which hole first? No matter what your answer, you'll find the equivalent expressions below. Just remember to stay safe and keep *Talk Dirty: French* next to your bedside so you'll be well-versed for round two . . .

coucher
to f**k, lit. to lay down
T'as vraiment couché avec cinquante mecs cet été?
Did you really f**k fifty guys this summer?

conclure
to have sex, lit. to conclude
Bastien était à deux doigts de conclure avec Ilona.
Bastien was very close to having sex with Ilona.

partie de jambes en l'air, f
roll between the sheets, lit. a game of legs in the air
Daniela est toujours d'accord pour une partie de jambes en l'air.
Daniela never says no to a roll between the sheets.

s'envoyer en l'air
to f**k, lit. to send oneself in the air
Ils s'envoient en l'air dans des endroits bizarres.
They f**k in strange places.

baiser
to f**k
Notre voisine baise toute la nuit.
Our neighbor f**ks all night long.

sauter
to f**k, lit. to jump
Thomas sauterait sur tout ce qui bouge.
Thomas would f**k anything that moves.

se taper qqn

to f**k somebody, lit. to hit someone oneself

Nathalie s'est tapée un inconnu dans le train.

Nathalie f**ked a stranger in the train.

tirer un coup avec qqn

to bang, lit. to shoot

Il est du genre à tirer un coup avec sa sœur sans demander la permission de leur mère.

He is the kind of person who would bang his sister without asking their mother's permission.

tremper le biscuit / le pinceau

to have sex, lit. to dip the biscuit / the brush

Si tu penses que tu peux tremper le biscuit au premier rencard, t'es bien naïf.

If you think you can have sex on the first date, you're out of your mind.

se faire qqn

to do someone

Ce soir, je mets le paquet pour me faire Virginie!

Tonight I'll do anything to do Virginie!

niquer

to f**k, to f**k up, abbr. of forniquer, to fornicate

Va niquer ta mère connard ou j'te nique la gueule!

Go f**k your mom, asshole, or I'll f**k up your face!

tringler

to f**k, to screw

T'aurais dû voir comment je l'ai tringlée ta voisine!

You should've seen how I screwed your neighbor!

graisser la queue
to f**k, lit. to lubricate the cock
Sam veut absolument graisser la queue ce soir.
Sam absolutely wants to f**k tonight.

planter la bitte à qqn
to f**k someone, lit. to plant
Il m'a planté sa bitte dans le cul, ce salaud.
He f**ked me in the ass, that bastard.

prendre par devant / derrière / tous les trous
to possess someone from in front, from behind, in every hole
Jeremy veut prendre Isabelle par derrière.
Jeremy wants to take Isabelle from behind.

prendre qqn en sandwich / en double
to have a (insert name) sandwich, lit. to take in sandwich, in
    double
Raoul et Rachid ont pris Djamileh en sandwich.
Raoul and Rachid had a Djamileh sandwich.

partouze, f
orgy, from party with the -ouze suffix
Chaque mois, ce club organise des partouzes géantes.
Every month, this club organizes a giant orgy.

cochonnerie, f
naughty things, from cochon, pig
Ils font des cochonneries dans ton appart!
They're doing naughty things in your flat.

aller à fond

to f**k deep, lit. to go to the edge
Il y est allé à fond, mais elle a aimé.
He f**ked her deep, but she liked it.

défoncer / démonter

to f**k hard, lit. to smash in / to take apart
Lance a défoncé Aline lors d'une soirée qui est partie en couille.
Lance f**ked Aline hard during a party that went out of control.

se faire baiser par tous les trous

to get f**ked in every hole
Melissa dit se faire régulièrement baiser par tous les trous.
XXX: Too Dirty to Translate

faire monter / descendre la température

to heat up / to cool off, lit. to make the temperature rise / fall
Toni est rentré avec une gonzesse hier, elle a vite fait monter la température en enlevant ses fringues.
Toni came back with a chick yesterday; she immediately made the temperature rise by taking off her clothes.

faire grimper aux rideaux

to come, lit. to climb the curtains
Nicolas peut faire grimper une miss au rideau rien qu'en la caressant.
XXX: Too Dirty to Translate

septième ciel, m

seventh heaven

**Après seulement dix minutes de baise avec Joey,
j'étais déjà au septième ciel.**

*Only ten minutes into f**king Joey, I was already in seventh
heaven.*

venir

to come

**Alizée était sur le point de venir quand Basile s'est
retiré.**

XXX: Too Dirty to Translate

balancer le foutre / la sauce

to ejaculate, to come, lit. to throw cum / the gravy

**T'aurais dû voir la tronche de ta cousine quand Steven
lui a balancé la sauce.**

XXX: Too Dirty to Translate

se cambrer

to bend over

Cambre-toi plus. J'vais te le carrer profond.

XXX: Too Dirty to Translate

à sec / à froid

without warming up, lit. dry/cold

Walter a essayé d'enculer à froid Jeffrey.

XXX: Too Dirty to Translate

BIBLIOGRAPHY

Deak, Etienne and Simone. *Dictionary of Colorful French Slanguage and Colloquialisms*. (New York, New York, USA: E P Dutton and Company Inc, 1961).

Edis, Geneviève. *The Complete Merde*. (London, Great Britain: HarperCollins Publishers, 1996).

Gagnière, Claude. *Tout sur Tout*. (Paris, France: France Loisirs, 1986).

Harrap, Chambers. *Harrap's Slang Dictionnaire*. (Edinburgh, Great Britain: Chambers Harrrap Publishers, 2007).

www.about.com

www.answers.com

www.argotnaut.fr

www.ask.com

www.coolslang.com

www.expressio.fr

www.ielanguages.com

www.languefrancaise.net

www.peevish.co.uk

www.slip-kangourou.tripod.com

www.wikipedia.com

www.worldreference.com